SHANG HAN LUN:
Wellspring of Chinese Medicine

Other Keats / OHAI Titles

SHANG HAN LUN:
Wellspring of Chinese Medicine

CHANG CHUNG-CHING
(A.D. 142-220)

with a modern interpretation by Otsuka Keisetsu

Edited by Hong-yen Hsu, Ph.D
& William G. Peacher, M.D.

Keats Publishing, Inc. ▓ New Canaan, Connecticut
Oriental Healing Arts Institute ◐ⓐ Long Beach, California

SHANG HAN LUN: WELLSPRING OF CHINESE MEDICINE

Copyright © 1981 by Oriental Healing Arts Institute

Keats Publishing edition published by arrangement with the Oriental Healing Arts Institute, Long Beach, California.

Library of Congress Cataloging-in-Publication Data

Chang, Chung-ching, fl.168-196.
   [Shang han lun. English & Chinese]
   Shang han lun : Wellspring of Chinese medicine / Chang
Chung-ching (A.D. 142-220), with a modern interpretation by
Otsuka Keisetsu ; edited by Hong-yen Hsu and Douglas
Peacher.
     p. cm.
   This edited and rev. ed. originally published: Long Beach,
Calif. Oriental Healing Arts Institute, 1981.
   Includes bibliographical references and index.
   ISBN 0-87983-669-5
   1. Medicine, Chinese—Early works to 1800. 2. Chang,
Chung-ching, fl. 168-196, Shang han lun. I. Hsu, Hung-yuan.
II. Peacher, William G., 1914- . III. Title.
R127.1.C42513 1995   95-1873
  615.8'99—dc20   CIP

Printed in the United States of America

Published by Keats Publishing, Inc.
27 Pine Street (Box 876)
New Canaan, Connecticut 06840-0876

98 97 96 95 6 5 4 3 2 1

Contents

PUBLISHER'S NOTE

Five years have been spent in translating and editing this book. The translation is taken from *Shang han lun chieh shuo* (傷寒論解說) written in Japanese by Otsuka Keisetsu (大塚敬節) in 1966, and *Shang han lun chuan shih* (傷寒論詮釋) written by Wu Kuo-ting (吳國定). In this book, detailed interpretations are printed alongside the original text of the *Shang han lun*. We have been able to include only the original text but hope to publish the work in its entirety at a later date. Handel Wu and Wang Su-yen with the assistance of Lu Yueh-ying did the translation for this edition. It was proofread and revised by Dr. Hsu Hong-yen, and Dr. Willian G. Peacher.

NOTICE

The detailed formulas in this book are put forth in an effort to be true to the original text. It is not intended that they be used for self-treatment.

The Publisher

PREFACE

In October of 1980 my father, Keisetsu Otsuka, passed away. When I learned that Dr. Hong-yen Hsu planned to publish an English version of my father's book, *The Interpretation of the Shang han lun for Clinical Application*, I was elated. I feel tremendous admiration for Dr. Hsu.

The *Shang han lun* (Treatise on Febrile Diseases) greatly influenced my father's life. In 1936 he happened upon a copy in a Tokyo bookstore. After carefully studying the book, he realized that the preface dated 1060, written by Tamba Masatata, a famous physician, indicated that it was a *Kang Ping* edition. It thus preceded Lin I's edition of the *Shang han lun* published in 1065 during the Sung dynasty. At that time, therefore, the *Kang Ping* edition must have been available in Japan, five years before the Sung edition was.

My father's book and teaching were based upon the *Kang Ping* edition. Because the *Shang han lun* combines theory and practice it remains a most important medical classic. For his book my father selected sections dealing with clinical application only and omitted those devoted to theory. In addition, my father added his own experiences to amplify his commentary.

The advent of this great classic in English is a most auspicious occasion. I am most grateful for Dr. Hsu's cooperation in overseeing the translation of this book. I hope that it will be widely accepted.

Yasuo Otsuka
Tokyo Japan,
September, 1981

LIST OF TABLES

FOREWORD

In China and Southeast Asia, where most overseas Chinese live, diseases are treated by Western as well as Chinese methods. Western therapy adopts an objective approach: first identifying the disease and its cause and then prescribing treatment specific to that condition. Chinese therapy, however, is subjective in that the patient's complaints and symptoms determine general treatment and there is no specific labeling of the disease. Western medicine emphasizes identification and specific treatment while Chinese medicine attempts to adjust imbalances in the system. In addition, the former uses mainly purified chemicals for drugs while the latter employs various herbs and natural materials. Although both aim to alleviate suffering, their theories and therapies vary considerably.

Western medicine has made great advancements in the diagnosis and treatment of disease. Nevertheless, there is much room for improvement in methods of treatment. For example, Western medicine has great difficulty in treating many diseases, such as hepatosis, diabetes mellitus, nephrosis, cardiopathies, rheumatism, hypertension, arteriosclerosis, allergies, female complaints, and cancer. Yet these same diseases can often be cured or the symptoms alleviated with Chinese herb medicine.

The medicinals used in Western medicine are either synthetic or extracts from natural materials. At the time of their discovery the therapeutic effects of certain drugs were manifest, and it was only gradually that their side effects became apparent: penicillin shock, thalidomide teratogenicity, and the side effects of prednisolone, an adrenal corticoid hormone. Due to the detrimental effects on the human body of many Western drugs, a re-evaluation of them has become necessary. In contrast, Chinese herbal medicine uses naturally occurring products for the treatment of disease. Although a few of these substances are potent poisons, most herbs are only slightly toxic. For this reason Chinese herbal therapy is growing in significance.

All countries have a native folk medicine that revolves around specific herbs used to treat certain diseases. However, most folk medicine is quite limited when compared to the Chinese medical tradition which represents a systematic and exhaustive effort to cope with the problem of health and disease. The latter bases its treatment on Chang Chung-ching's *Shang han lun* (傷寒論), a book more than eighteen hundred years old. The therapeutic methods and herbs recorded therein are still being used today. No other Chinese medical classic rivals the *Shang han lun* (傷寒論) in having so many commentaries and research books written about it. Moreover, in recent years study of the *Shang han lun* has increased in Southeast Asian countries, especially Japan. This not only demonstrates its importance but also indicates that interpretations vary. According to Takino Kazuo's second report appearing in the *Journal of the Oriental Medical Society of Japan* (日本東洋醫學會誌), there are as many as 531 written works on the *Shang han lun* in Japanese literature alone. Dr. Keisetsu cites forty well-known books in his book *The Interpretation of the Shang han lun for Clinical Application* (臨床應用傷寒論解說). In China no one can be certain as to how many works have been written on the *Shang han lun*, but it is believed that the number might well be over one thousand. In Japan the famous physician Kondai Wutsuki (宇津木昆臺) of the Tokugawa period bestowed these admiring words on the *Shang han lun*: "Never before has there been such a wonderful work as this. Who else except a sage could write it?" Many Japanese men of wisdom have remarked that without the *Shang han lun* there would be no Chinese medicine. The *Shang han lun* is to Chinese medicine what the *Analects of Confucius* (論語) and the *Works of Mencius* (孟子) are to Confucianism.

At the time of the writing of the *Shang han lun*, the art of printing was not well developed; hence no one is sure of the actual form of the original. Presently, the following versions of the *Shang han lun* are available:

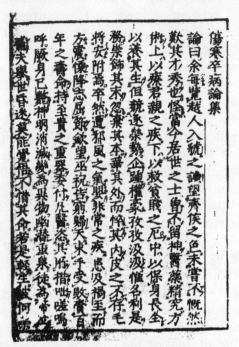

The beginning part of the foreword of the Sung edition
Shang han lun

1. Sung edition of the *Shang han lun* (宋板傷寒論). This edition was collated by the scholastic ministers Kao Pao-hen, Lin I, and Sun Chi under the order of the emperor and published in 1065. Regarded as a national textbook, the original nevertheless disappeared for a long time. The Sung edition that we have today is a reprint by Chao Kai-mei of the Ming dynasty. It is beautifully worded and always has been highly respected by annotators.

2. Cheng Wu-chi's *Annotated Shang han lun* (成無己註解傷寒論). This version of the *Shang han lun* was extensively read in Japan and China and was widely circulated in Cheng's time. However, many transcriptions and retranscriptions have stirred up disagreement as to whether this is true to the original.

3. *Chin kuei yu han ching* (金匱玉函經). This book has the same content as the Sung edition with only minor variations in context.

4. Kang Ping edition of the *Shang han lun* (康平傷寒論).

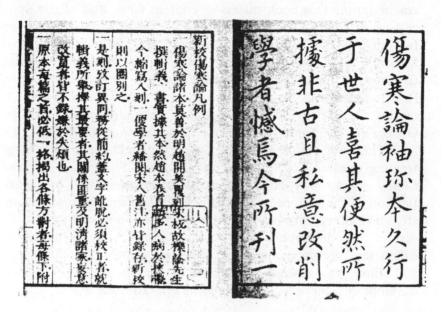

Parts of the foreword and the general notices of the Sung edition *New Collated Shang han lun*

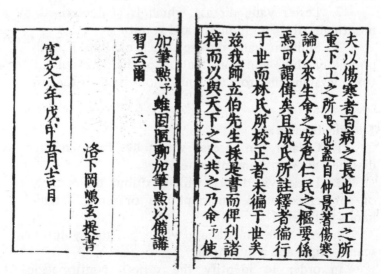

The epigraph in the firstly published *Shang han lun* in Japan.

Kang Ping is the name of the period from 1058-1068 in the Heian era in Japan. This book differs in content from that of the Sung edition or Cheng's edition of *Shang han lun* in that it lacks the two chapters on "Pulse Identification" and "Pulses in a Normal Person." The work is done in three different styles, namely, fifteen-word lines, fourteen-word lines, and thirteen-word lines. It is indispensable for the study of the *Shang han lun* because it retains the ancient style. The text of this edition was used by Otsuka Keisetsu for *A Study of the Shang han lun* (傷寒論解説).

The chief contribution of Chang Chung-ching is his way of treating diseases which he recorded in the *Shang han lun* and *Chin kuei yao lueh*. His methods of therapy are based on identification of the various confirmations. (A confirmation is the constellation of symptoms, plus the treatment required.) First, he divided the development of diseases into six stages which he called the "six proceedings" of illnesses, namely, the three yang and three yin diseases. For each of the six stages of disease development, there are corresponding prescriptions.

The yang diseases are:

1. Greater yang disease which exhibits the main symptoms of buoyant pulse, headache, fever, and chills.

2. Lesser yang disease which is characterized by a bitter mouth, dry throat, giddiness, and vomiting.

3. Sunlight yang disease which exhibits periods of anemophobia or chills and constipation or diarrhea due to the disease toxin invading the stomach and various parts of the viscera.

The yin diseases are:

1. Greater yin disease which has the main symptoms of diarrhea, vomiting, and dysentery.

2. Lesser yin disease which exhibits the cardinal symptoms of submerged pulse, anemophobia or chills, fatigue, and cold hands and feet.

3. Absolute yin disease which has the symptoms of thirst, scanty urine, and exhaustion.

In order to identify the various confirmations, Chinese medicine employs four methods of diagnosis: "observation," "listening and smelling," "inquiry," and "palpation." These four methods can be explained briefly as follows:

Observation
The doctor notes the patient's external appearance with his eyes. If the patient has a robust physique and good nutrition, he has a firm confirmation; whereas if the patient has a delicate and slender physique, pale complexion, frail and thin skeleton, and little strength, he has a weak confirmation. Diagnosis is then made by observing the physique, complexion, and condition and color of the nails, lips, and eyes.

Listening and Smelling
The doctor further detects the patient's confirmation by listening for coughs, gasping, and length and frequency of respiration and by registering odors of the mouth and body.

Inquiry
The doctor questions the patient concerning his complaints, such as chillphobia, anemophobia, fever, perspiration, thirst, dry throat, headache, vertigo, tinnitus, conditions relating to urine and stools, vomiting, abdominal aches, chest pains, edema, appetite, and so on.

Palpation
The doctor feels the pulse and abdomen. In pulse palpating the doctor presses his fingers on the radial arterial pulses of the patient and from the buoyancy or submergency, slowness or quickness, longness or shortness, tightness or slackness of the beat determines whether the patient's confirmation is superficial or internal, weak or firm, cold or hot. In abdominal palpating the physician presses the patient's abdomen to test the elasticity and reaction from which he tells once again whether the patient's confirmation is weak or firm.

The above four methods of diagnosis are done collectively to decide upon treatment. Such means of diagnosis for diseases have been employed in the Orient for a very long time but are little known to the West. Also in the Orient, annotative books on the *Shang han lun* are in the thousands while in the West there is not even the most fundamental translation.

The Oriental Healing Arts Institute of the United States has been established to accelerate the introduction of the theories and practical application of Chinese herbal medicine to the West. To do so, this institute publishes bulletins on Chinese herb medicine at regular intervals and translates the more important Chinese medical classics.

After more than two years of translation and compilation, we are finally ready to present this book to the reader. The following references were used to compile this edition.

1. *The Explanation of the Shang han lun* (吳國定傷寒論 詮釋) by Wu Kuo-ting, professor of the China Medical College. This book is based on an original Sung edition of the *Shang han lun*—Taki Genkan's *Shang han lun chi i* (多紀元簡著傷寒論輯義 A Compendium of the Meaning of *Shang han lun*). (Extensive annotations ought to be added to the main text of our translation; however, owing to the limitation in time, these notes will be appended to the second edition.) In the present translation, the Chinese original is printed alongside the English version to facilitate the reader's comprehension of the original meaning. A translation of parts of this work is in the Biographical Notes.

2. To help the reader understand the background of the *Shang han lun*, we have also included "The Comprehension" (the commentaries) part from *A Study of the Shang han lun* (傷寒論 解說) by Otsuka Keisetsu, a great scholar of Chinese herb medicine in Japan and director of Oriental Medicine Research Center of the Kitasato Institute.

3. The Introduction was contributed by Dr. William G. Peacher, a noted neurologist and neurosurgeon who has been interested in and has studied Chinese herbal medicine for some years.

Never before has a complete English translation of the *Shang han lun* been published, and it would give the translator great pleasure and honor if the publication of this book should arouse in the Western world an interest in furthering Oriental medical science. This book is divided into two parts: the commentaries and the main text. They were translated by Hendel Wu and Wang Su-yen respectively with the assistance of Miss Lu Yueh-

ying. All translations were edited and revised by Dr. William G.
Peacher and Ms. Judith Haueter with the assistance of staff
members of the Oriental Healing Arts Institute. It was proofread
by Miss Lu Yueh-ying and Miss Wang Su-kuei. I am deeply
indebted to all of them for their unstinting efforts in bringing
this work to fruition.

Hong-yen Hsu, Ph.D.,
President
Oriental Healing Arts Institute of the United States

INTRODUCTION

This is the fourth volume on the history, development, and pharmacology of Chinese medicine that I have had the privilege of collaborating on with Dr. Hong-yen Hsu. The three earlier works were *Chinese Herb Medicine and Therapy, Chen's History of Chinese Medical Science, and How to Treat Yourself with Chinese Herbs*, all published by the Oriental Healing Arts Institute of the U.S.A.

This fourth work is the first English translation of the Chinese medical classic *Shang han lun*, together with pertinent and significant translations of several commentaries from the original Chinese or Japanese. A brief review of Chinese medicine in the Han dynasty is relevant to our study.

Dual concepts that underlay the development of medicine in Han China (206 B.C.-A.D. 221) can be seen as (1) an official medicine based on natural philosophical tenets with rational qualities that was part of the scholarly world of Confucius; and (2) a popular medicine with strong magico-religious elements chiefly based in Taoism.

Early Chinese medicine revolved around five focal points: the philosophical principles of yin-yang and the Five Elements; *Huang ti nei ching* (黃帝內經), a book on acupuncture; *Shang han lun* (傷寒論), a book of prescription formulas used for the treatment of febrile and other diseases; *Shen nung pen ts'ao ching* (神農本草經), a materia medica or description of drugs; and Chinese folk medicine.

The following aspects of medicine are being practiced

RIGHT—Sheng Nung, c. 3494 B.C., is the Chinese God of Husbandry. From a wood carving.
(Also Shen Nung.)

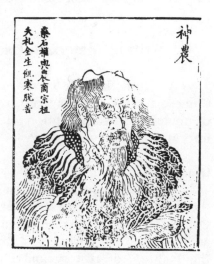

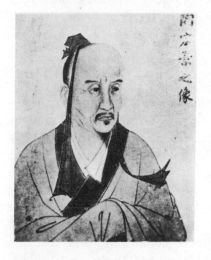

LEFT-Tao Hung-Ching, A.D. 452-536, collected ancient records for *The Book on Herbs by Sheng Nung.* His greatest contribution was his study of herbs.

throughout the Orient today: shamanism, divination, fortune telling, physiognomy, traditional medicine, and modern medicine. Traditional medicine has always recognized a wide variety of illnesses. As a medical practice, it functions primarily in the field of internal medicine.

The *Shu ching* (書經 Book of Odes) compiled by unknown authors during the Chou period (ninth to fifth centuries B.C.) first discussed natural medicinals. Then came the *Shan hai ching* (山海經 Classic of the Mountain and Sea). It was divided into two sections which were compiled at two different times, the Shan ca. 400 B.C. and the Hai ca. 250 B.C. The *Shan ching* (山經) is a geography of China, particularly of the mountain ranges. Twenty-six chapters mention medicine. The various descriptions include 270 animals, 70 minerals, and 150 plants. Of these, 47 animal and 21 plant parts were used in the treatment of disease. Some examples are realgar, talc, dragon bone, bos, cinnamon, *tang-kuei*, cnidium, and platycodon. There is no medical data in the *Hai ching* (海經), the second section. The entire work has been translated recently by Chen Cheng-hui.

Writing Materials Used in Ancient China

At least eight different media were used by the ancient Chinese for the written word. (See Table I for dates and types of materials.) A description of each material and the medical information conveyed follows.

Oracle Bones (Chia-ku Wen 甲骨文)

Inscriptions on tortoise shells and animal bones, commonly the scapula, appear to be the earliest known form of writing in China. They were discovered in 1899. Considerable subsequent archeological field work and research is being carried out by the Institute of History and Philology of the Academia Sinica at the Hsin-tun village (site of the capital of the Yin dynasty) in An Yang in Honan Province. As could be anticipated for this era, the markings were concerned largely with divination. No herbs were mentioned but some medical conditions were described: scabies, blindness, childhood conditions, and diseased body parts, such as the foot, hand, eye, ear, tooth, and tongue. There are representative exhibits of these oracle bones at the National Palace Museum and the Museum of the Academia Sinica in Taipei, Taiwan. For additional information on this subject see Chapter 3 in our revision of *Chen's History of Chinese Medicine*, 1977, and the article "Chinese Oracle Bones" in the *Scientific American*, April 1979.

Bamboo and Wooden Slips

Archeological investigation in December 1972 in Wu Wei County, Kansu Province P.R.C., uncovered 92 inscribed wooden (pine or poplar) slips attributed to the early Eastern Han dynasty (A.D. 25-220). There are more than thirty prescriptions written down concerning internal medicine, surgery, gynecology, and eye, ear, nose, throat, oral, and dental problems. Some of the conditions treated were fevers, diseases of the various systems—circulatory, respiratory, digestive, nervous, and genitourinary—ulcers,

Table I
Writing Materials Used in Ancient China

Writing Material	Dynasty	Dates
oracle bones	Shang (Yin)	1765-1123 B.C.
bronze	Western Chou	1122-771 B.C.
silk	Eastern Chou	770-256 B.C.
silk	Ch'un Ch'iu	722-481 B.C.
bamboo, wood	Chan Kuo	468-221 B.C.
stone	Ch'in	221-202 B.C.
quasi-paper	Former Han	206 B.C.-A.D. 8
true paper	Later Han	A.D. 25-220

carbuncles, dog bites, urinary calculi, deafness, dental diseases, and nasal polyps. The prescriptions include the name of the disease, symptoms, nature, cause, medication to be used—its preparation, dosage, method of administration, and contraindications. Acupuncture and moxibustion were discussed including indication, techniques, and the names and locations of certain points and forbidden areas. One hundred different medicaments from the vegetable (61), mineral (16), and animal (11) kingdoms are described. Most of these are still used as ingredients of prescriptions today.

Six hundred and ten bamboo strips were discovered in Tomb No. 3 of the Western Han dynasty at Mawangtui, a suburb of Changsha, Hunan Province, P.R.C., in 1973-1974. Two hundred of them contain a medical essay written in a style similar to the *Huang ti nei ching* (黃帝內經 Yellow Emperor's Classic of Internal Medicine) and to the *Huang ti wai ching* (黃帝外經) of which no known copy is extant.

Further information on these bamboo and wooden slips can be found in Chapter 4 of *Chen's History of Chinese Medicine* (陳存仁中國醫學史), 1977.

Writings on Silk

Numerous medical writings on silk were discovered in the same tomb with the wooden slips previously discussed. These include essays on moxibustion, pulse diagnosis, fasting and breathing exercises, diagnosis of the symptoms of diseases, and a drawing called "Illustrated Gymnastics." There are also 270 prescriptions with dosage listed, plus the methods of treatment for 52 various diseases and conditions.

The corpse of the wife of the Marquis of Tai was found in Tomb No. 1 at Mawangtui. An autopsy was performed with interesting results but not pertinent to the present discussion. Six silk pouches were also discovered during the excavations. They contained herbal medicine such as magnolia bark, sweet grass, cinnamon, lesser galangal, prickly ash seeds, and cayenne pepper.

Literature

The significance of these archeological finds is apparent as they represent the earliest known medical works in their original forms. Unfortunately, the surviving well-known Chinese medical classics *Huang ti nei ching* (黃帝內經), *Nan ching* (難經), *Shen nung pen ts'ao ching* (神農本草經), and *Shang han lun* (傷寒論) discussed in this preface do not exist in their original forms and have suffered from frequent revisions and alterations by many physicians through the succeeding ages.

The first Chinese herbal, known as the *Shen nung pen ts'ao ching*, is no longer extant. It is associated with the Western Han dynasty (206 B.C.-A.D. 25) and represented a compilation of all the then known herbs (365). Although ascribed to Shan Nung, a legendary emperor who ruled 2838-2698 B.C., it was actually written by various unknown authors (Fang-shih). The herbs were classified as follows:

1. Upper rank, 120 herbs to nourish life
2. Middle rank, 120 herbs to supplement nature
3. Lower rank, 125 herbs to cure disease

The earliest surviving herbal was written by Tao Hung-ching (A.D. 452-536) with the title of *Shen nung pen ts'ao ching*. It includes a discussion of the 365 different herbs originally attributed to Shen Nung. Tao Hung-ching later added a supplement to this work entitled *Ming i pieh lu* (名醫別錄) which covered 365 more herbs used by well-known physicians in the Han and Wei dynasties. Both volumes were then combined with a commentary under the name of *Pen ts'ao ching chi chu* (本草經集註). This study could rightly be termed the first commentary on Chinese materia medica.

The *Huang ti nei ching*, the oldest and one of the most

important Chinese medical texts, is an anthology of material compiled by unknown authors in the early Han dynasty. Some investigators, however, have attributed its origin to the period of the Warring States (403-206 B.C.). It is based upon contemporary philosophical concepts interwoven into a system of internal medicine. The book describes an energy or *ch'i* quality of internal organs; reviews anatomy, physiology, and hygiene; classifies symptoms and signs of disease; and delineates the proper administration of therapy, either acupuncture, moxibustion, or massage. There was very little on the use of herbs. The theory of the five elements with their geographical correlations, the four methods of diagnosis, the *ching-lo* (經絡 meridians), and the eight rubrics were integral parts of this medical system.

It is interesting that these classical medical theories appeared in written form about the same time that Hippocrates, the father of Western medicine, wrote his 87 essays on medicine.

The earliest reference to the *Nei ching* is in Pan Ku's catalogue of the main contents of the Imperial Library compiled at the end of the first century B.C. The *Nei ching* appeared in *History of the Former Han Dynasty* (206 B.C.-A.D. 25). The notation said, "*Huang ti nei ching*: 18 rolls; *Huang ti wai ching*: 37 rolls."

It is interesting that this work was referred to by Chang Chung-ching (A.D. 142-220) in the *Shang han lun*. Huang Fu-mi (A.D. 215-282) mentioned it also in the preface of his work *Chia i ching* (甲乙經). The full title *Huang ti nei ching su wen* (黃帝內經素問) was not used until the *Annals* of the Sui dynasty (A.D. 589-618) when only eight volumes were listed.

Wang Ping of the T'ang dynasty said that he had received a copy of the original edition belonging to Chang Chung-ching from his teacher Kuo Tzu-chai. On completing his edition of this great work in A.D. 762, he wrote a preface to it indicating that he had combined the former with all available material and expanded the original into 24 books divided into 81 chapters. This, therefore, represents the main book as we know it today.

Kao Pao-heng and Lin I, based on Wang Ping's earlier edition, rearranged and revised the text from A.D. 1068-1078 during the reign of Shen Tsung of the Sung dynasty.

The *Nei ching* has been discussed and reviewed by many investigators through the centuries. It has been widely re-edited with commentaries in Chinese and other Oriental languages, notably Japanese. It is only in this century that efforts have been made to make the original text available to the Western world.

Ilza Veith translated the first 34 chapters of the *Nei ching* into English in 1949; this version has been reprinted in recent years.

A. Chamfrault with Kang-sam Ung rendered the entire work into French in 1957 under the title *Les livres sacres de medecine chinoise.* This is Volume 2 of Chamfrault's five volume work on *Traite de medecine chinoise 1957-1964.*

Henry C. Lu is currently translating the *Nei ching* (four volumes) and *Nan ching* (one volume) into English. The *Su wen* (素問) in two volumes has already been published, and the *Ling shu* (靈樞) also in two volumes will appear at a later date.

Robert Banever is now transcribing a Vietnamese edition of the *Nei ching* into English.

An outline summary of the *Nei ching* in English was completed by Wong Man and published in the *Chinese Medical Journal*, Volume 68, pages 1-33, in 1950.

The *Nan ching* (Difficult Classic or the Book on Medical Perplexities) appeared in the Han dynasty. It has been attributed to Pien Ch'iao (Chin Yueh-jen) ca. 407-310 B.C. It consists primarily of an explanation of 81 difficult passages from the *Nei ching.* Perhaps the most useful existing edition was completed by Hua Shou in the Yuan dynasty and is called *Nan ching pen i* (難經本義). An equally popular version was written by Chang Shih-hsien during the reign of Ching To (A.D. 1506-1521) in the Ming dynasty. This has been translated into German by F. Hubotter and is currently being translated into English by Henry C. Lu.

The importance of Chang Chung-ching's contribution to medical science and thought cannot be overemphasized. Besides his monumental work the *Shang han lun* on the symptoms and treatment of febrile diseases, he was the first to separate illnesses into the three yang and the three yin categories. His second work *Chin kuei yao lueh* reviews many conditions, such as those of the digestive tract, nephrosis, rheumatism, and gynecological problems. This will be the subject of a subsequent translation.

The *Shang han lun* represented a new system of medicine. Disease manifestations were classified within the yin-yang system according to its six stages, and the *ching-lo* were also integrated within this framework. Although some useful acupuncture and moxibustion points were included, the main therapeutic emphasis was on herbal prescriptions.

There are many early references citing the value of this work. Hua To (A.D. 110-207), the father of Chinese surgery and pioneer in anesthesia (*Ma-fei-san* or Indian hemp was used for surgery), described it as a "real life-saving book." Huang Fu-mi (A.D. 215-286), author of the *Chia i ching* (甲乙經), the earliest surviving work on acupuncture, said that "most of the remedies recommended were very effective." Tao Hung-ching (A.D. 452-536), a well-known Taoist of the Liang dynasty who compiled *Ming i pieh lu* (Formulas of Famous Physicians) based on the earlier *Shen nung pen ts'ao ching*, wrote, "Chang Chung-ching's book was the first book of therapy." Sun Szu-mo (A.D. 590-682), a noted herbal physician and author of two popular medical works in the T'ang dynasty—*Pei chi chien chin yao fang* (備急千金要方 Precious Formulas for Emergency) and *Chien chin i fang* (千金翼方 Precious Supplementary Formulas)—also described Chang's investigations as most profound and useful.

Wong and Wu (*History of Chinese Medicine*, 1932) said the *Shang han lun* is to medicine what the "Four Classics" are to philosophy, the "Four Classics" being *Lun yu* (論語 Digested Conversations: Sayings of Confucius or Confucian Analects); *Ta hsiao* (大學 Great Learning) commonly attributed to Tsang Shan, a disciple of Confucius; *Chung yung* (中庸 Doctrine of the Means) ascribed to K'ung Chi, grandson of Confucius; and the *Works of Mencius* (孟子). Accordingly *Huang ti nei ching* compares with the "Five Classics": *I ching* (易經 The Book of Changes); *Shu ching* (書經 The Book of History); *Shih ching* (詩經 The Book of Poetry); *Li chi* (禮記 The Record of Rites); and *Ch'un ch'iu* (春秋 Spring and Autumn).

Yasuo Otsuko in his recent article "Chinese Traditional Medicine in Japan" (*Asian Medical Systems*, pages 322-340, 1976) said that the *Shang han lun* contains 113 prescriptions and *Chin kuei yao lueh*, 262. Since a great many of these formulas are still used effectively, these two works are not only important classics for medical historians but also indispensable textbooks for contemporary medical practitioners. In fact, Chinese traditional medicine continues to be very popular and widely practical throughout the Orient today.

Manfred Porkert in his paper "The Intellectual and Social Impulses Behind the Evolution of Traditional Chinese Medicine" in *Asian Medical Systems*, pages 63-76, 1976, said, "*Shang han tsa ping lun* (傷寒雜病論 Shang han lun) may be called the first clinical manual in Chinese medical literature, and it has become the classic text on clinical medicine throughout the sphere of Chinese culture."

Medical literature in English relating to Chinese medicine has been thoroughly searched relative to any possible translation of the *Shang han lun* with negative results. Dr. Hsu has also reviewed the Oriental literature in this respect with similar findings. I corresponded with several of the librarians of some of the larger libraries in the United States that have extensive Chinese collections and came to the same conclusion. These included:

Mrs. Iping King Wei, administrative assistant to the curator, and Ms. Maureen Donovan, reference librarian of the Gest Oriental Library and East Asian Collections, Princeton University Library, Princeton, New Jersey.

Chi Wang, head of the Chinese and Korean section of the Library of Congress, Washington, D.C.

Edith D. Blair, head of the reference section of the Reference Services Division, National Library of Medicine, National Institute of Health, Bethesda, Maryland.

Thomas G. Falio, assistant historical librarian of the Historical Library, Yale Medical Library, New Haven, Connecticut.

As of June 13, 1977, my last correspondence with them, none of these prestigious libraries had an English version of the *Shang han lun*.

There are no copies of the *Shang han lun* in the libraries at Gest Chinese Research Library at McGill University, Montreal, Quebec; the Chinese Library of Columbia University, New York City, New York; John Crerar Library, Chicago, Illinois; Harvard University, Cambridge, Massachusetts; or the University of California, Berkeley, California.

Some of the problems that exist for the Western scholar in identifying with Chinese medicine have been discussed by Porkert in his book *Medicine in Chinese Culture* published in 1975. He emphasized that in order for the Western investigator to completely understand traditional Chinese and modern medicine he must have knowledge of four separate disciplines. He must

1. Be conversant with Chinese philology

2. Be thoroughly familiar with the Chinese medical classics *Nei ching, Shang han lun,* and *Pen ts'ao*

3. Know the various scientific methods as defined in the West, and

4. Be widely acquainted with various medical procedures and problems.

He must also

5. Be familiar with the Chinese culture and the classics: the "Four Books" and the "Five *Ching*" mentioned above, and

6. Be aware of the development of Chinese traditional medicine to modern times.

William G. Peacher, M.D.

Biographical Notes on Chang
Chung-ching

Chang Chung-ching—also known as Chi, Chang-chi and Chung Ching—was the most prominent medical practitioner of the Later Han dynasty (A.D. 142-220). In fact, he is one of the most celebrated of all Chinese physicians, venerated through the centuries as the Sage of Medicine and often referred to as the Chinese Hippocrates. It is indeed fortunate that his immortal work, a landmark in the history of medicine, has survived the ravages of time. It has served countless generations as the basis of diagnosis and treatment in traditional Chinese medicine. It remains as popular and useful today as when it was written, is readily available in numerous translations at any bookstore specializing in works printed in Oriental languages, and ranks on a plane with the better known, ancient and legendary medical classic *Huang ti nei ching* (黃帝內經 The Yellow Emperor's Classic of Internal Medicine). Chang's writings were published originally as a single work bearing the title *Shang han tsa ping lun* (傷寒卒 病論 Manual on Febrile and Miscellaneous Diseases) and only later subdivided into two separate works: *Shang han lun* (傷寒論 Manual on Febrile Diseases) and *Chin kuei yao lueh* (金匱要略 Synopsis of the Golden Chamber). In these treatises, he endorsed therapy by means of established formulas, described the rules of treatment by confirmation, and elaborated on the subdivisions of yin and yang and their importance in the diagnosis and management of various types of illnesses.

It is unfortunate that the Han annals, replete with information relating to the significant leaders and scholars of the period,

RIGHT—Chang Chung-Ching, A.D. 142-220, probably the world's first medical specialist, established the Chinese formula therapy during the Latter Han Dynasty. From his portrait in the collection of the Imperial Palace.

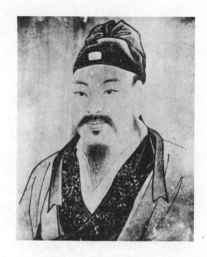

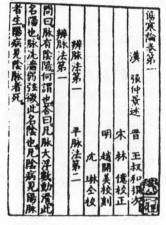

LEFT—From Chang's book, *Shang han lun*

fail to include his name. We are, therefore, dependent upon secondary resources for information about him, such as data collected by Lee Chiu-chih, et al.

The original *Shang han tsa ping lun* (傷寒雜病論) which appeared in A.D. 217 has been lost. We are indebted to Wang Su-ho (A.D. 265-317), the well-known authority on the pulse who wrote *Mo ching* (脈經 The Pulse Classic), for his efforts in preserving and collecting all available material on the *Shang han lun* (傷寒論) and publishing it in a work of ten volumes.

Chang Chung-ching's decision to practice medicine was prompted by the death of many of the members of his family from the severe epidemics which raged at that time in the Ching Chou province. This is fully attested to by his remarks in the "Preface" of the *Shang han lun* (傷寒論).

During the first ten years of the Chien-an era (A.D. 196) of the Later Han dynasty, two-thirds of my relatives [consisting] of more than two hundred members succumbed to disease, seven-tenths of which [deaths] were due to epidemic fever. [For this reason and] in consideration of [all those] lost and not saved in the past, I decided to seek diligently the ancient instruction and [accordingly] adopt various well-known formulas.

Stimulated by this great tragedy and in spite of being greatly depressed and lonely, he assiduously studied the ravaging effect of febrile and other diseases, collected formulas and reviewed all available previous works, and finally completed his immortal work *Shang han tsa ping lun* (傷寒雜病論) which inspires and aids students of Chinese medicine to this day.

There has been much debate over the original form of this book. According to Chang's own preface (q.v.) the work was entitled *Shang han tsa ping lun* (傷寒雜病論) and consisted of 16 volumes. The standard bibliographies are silent on this point. *The Annals of Literature of the Sui Dynasty* (隋書經籍志) (A.D. 589-618), however, states that Chang Chung-ching's work consisted of ten volumes. *The Annals of Art of the New T'ang Dynasty* (新唐書藝文志) (A.D. 618-907) lists one book bearing the title *Shang han tsa ping lun*(傷寒雜病論)in ten volumes. The *Shang han lun*(傷寒論) in ten volumes is also recorded in *The Annals of Art of the Sung Dynasty* (宋史藝文志)(A.D. 960-1278). This later work represents the *Shang han lun* (傷寒論) as we know it today.

From a study of the available sources, it would appear that the treatise actually did exist as its author indicated in sixteen volumes under the composite title of *Shang han tsa ping lun* (傷寒雜病論);then later under the editorship of Wang Su-ho (A.D. 210-285), it was separated into two sections: *Shang han lun* (傷寒論) in ten volumes, which covered all epidemic and endemic febrile illnesses and *Chin kuei yao lueh*(金匱要略)in six volumes, which included discussion of the diagnosis and treatment of diseases of the various body systems—digestive, respiratory, genitourinary, obstetrical, gynecological, and nervous.

Wang Su-ho's rendition of the original has been criticized unjustly through the centuries. Certainly, as to time, he was in the best situation to examine and evaluate the existing material since he lived in the generation succeeding that of the author and preceding that of his critics who wrote centuries later. One of these men, Fang Chung-hang (A.D. 1580), disputed Wang's arrangement of the material in his book *Shang han lun tiao pien* (傷寒論條辨 Discussion of the *Shang han lun*). Yu Chia-yin continued the argument in *Shang han lun tiao pien*(傷寒論條辨) (Discussion of the *Shang han lun*) and in *Shang han lun chung p'ien* (傷寒論重編 Essay on Infectious Diseases Re-edited) published ca. 1853. The dispute was further augmented by Cheng Chiao-ching in his somewhat unethical *Shang han hou tiao p'ien* (More Discussion of the *Shang han lun*). Fortunately, none of these later works ever erased the valuable contribution made by Wang and in fact did much to stimulate numerous interesting and significant commentaries.

Perhaps the best edition of the *Shang han lun* (傷寒論) now in existence was compiled by Cheng Wu-i in the Chin dynasty (A.D. 265-420). Ten of the fourteen volumes represent the original text as compiled by Wang Su-ho with the remaining four being done by Cheng. This edition consists of 22 essays, 397 rules for the treatment of disease, and 113 prescriptions which include small numbers of potent herbs rather than extensive formulas. Two of Chang's favorite herbs, cinnamon and bupleurum, formed the basis of many of his prescriptions. He also discussed the use of herbs and cold water for febrile illness and the application and value of the sweating method. Chang was one of the early proponents of use of enemas.

The second part, *Chin kuei yao lueh* (金匱要略), covers miscellaneous diseases and is somewhat less well known than the *Shang han lun* (傷寒論). The most useful edition was done by Hsu Pin of the Ch'ing dynasty. This work is in the process of being translated into English.

Other less significant works attributed to Chang Chung-ching but now lost are

1. *Huang Su Prescriptions* (皇叔方): twenty-five volumes
2. *Treatment of Diseases of the Cold* (傷寒療法 *Typhoid Fever Remedies*): one volume
3. *Diagnostic Methods* (診斷法): two volumes
4. *Prescriptions for Women's Diseases* (婦人病處方): two volumes
5. *Chang Chung-ching's Prescriptions* (張仲景方):fifteen volumes and the following consisting of one volume each
6. *The Pulse Classic* (脈經)
7. *Essay on Nutrition of the Five Organs* (五官營養論)
8. *Essay on the Five Organs* (五官論)
9. *The Book on the Treatment of Yellow Diseases* (黃疸療法 *On the Treatment of Jaundice*)
10. *Essay on the Teeth and Mouth* (論牙與嘴)

Birthplace of Chang Chung-ching

Although current opinion has it that Chang Chung-ching was born in Nan Yang, early records present conflicting evidence. The *Biographical Encyclopedia of Honan Province* (河南通志) says that he was a native of Nieh Yang whereas Lu Chiu-chih in his *Biography of Chang Chung-ching* (張仲景傳) says he was born in Nieh Yang, Nan Chun. Huang Chien in his *Biography of Chang Chung-ching* (張仲景傳) lists him as a native of Chi Yang, Nan Yang. Finally, the *Dictionary of Famous Chinese Persons* (published by Commercial Press, Ltd.) says he was a native of Chao Yang. We, therefore, have several possible places of birth: Nan Yang, Nan Chun, Nieh Yang, and Chao Yang. A further explanation is necessary. Geographically, Nan Yang and Nan Chun are different regions and should not be confused. There were thirty-six counties (*hsien*) under the legislative sanction of the Nan Yang district, situated in the southwest part of Honan province and the northern sector of Hupei. The Nan Chun region consisted of eighteen counties (*hsien*) located in the west-central section of Hupei province.

Perhaps one of the most convincing references in favor of Chang's birth in Nan Yang appears in the *Geographical and Administrative Record of the Later Han Dynasty* in the biography of Ho Yu. It states that Ho Yu and Chang Chung-ching were natives of Hsiang Yang in the Nan Yang district and friends from childhood.

Question of Serving as Governor of Changsha

Although Chang Chung-ching holds a distinguished position in Chinese medical history, his personal life has been shrouded in mystery. Few facts can be gleaned from historical sources with no records extant concerning his birth and death. It is extremely doubtful that he ever served as governor of Changsha, Honan province, although legend has accorded him this honor. The foundation for this concept was no doubt laid in the suggestion of this possibility in *Li tai ming i hsing ming* (歷代名醫姓名 The Biographies of Famous Physicians) by Kan Po-tsung in the T'ang dynasty (A.D. 618-907). At that time, no one seemed to question the authenticity of his having been the governor of

Changsha. Doubt was first cast upon this assumption by Ting Fu-pao in his *Li tai ming i chuan* (歷代名醫傳 Biographies of Famous Physicians of the Ages) in which he remarked that Chang's name did not appear in the list of governors of Changsha during the reigns of any of the emperors of the Later Han dynasty.

Copies of the *Shang han lun* (傷寒論) published in Japan during the Sung dynasty (A.D. 960-1280) in referring to the author state simply, "Dictated by Chang Chung-ching, Han dynasty." Further, there is no reference to his having been governor in the edition published by Chao Kai-mei during the Ming dynasty (A.D. 1368-1644). Cheng's rendition reads, "Written by Chang Chung-ching, Han dynasty." Searches through many versions of the *Chin kuei yao lueh* (金匱要略) have cast no further light on this subject. It would appear, therefore, that we have no basis to substantiate the fact that Chang ever served in an official government capacity. It would seem that this myth was fabricated by Kan Po-tsung or others in the T'ang dynasty.

Education

The evidence that Chang Chung-ching received his medical education from Chang Po-tsu of Nan Yang is based on a statement recorded by Kan Po-tsung in *Li tai ming i hsing ming* (歷代名醫 姓名) which appeared in the T'ang dynasty. Subsequent records have been based upon Kan's declaration.

Chang Kuo in the Sung dynasty (A.D. 960-1280) stated in *I shuo* (醫說) (Chang's Medical Talks):

Chang Po-tsu of Nan Yang was a quiet, simple, and skillful physician, careful in diagnosis and successful in treatment. He was held in great esteem by the community. Chang Chung-ching of the same region respected him greatly and learned medicine from him. Because of this Chang Chung-ching became established as a man of reputation.

Ku chin i yao chuan shu (古今醫藥纂述 The Complete Work of Ancient and Modern Medicines) written by Hsu Dhun-pu of the Ming dynasty (A.D. 1368-1644), states:

Chang Po-tsu, a native of Nan Yang, was very fond of studying medical classics and skillful in taking the pulse and accomplished in therapy. He was held in high esteem by the people and taught Chang Chung-ching medicine.

Lu Chiu-chih of the Ch'ing dynasty (A.D. 1644-1911) in his *Hou han shu chang chung-ching chuan pu i* (後漢書張仲景傳補遺 Supplement to Chang Chi's Biography in the Later Han Records) cites, "Chang Chung-ching learned medicine from Chang Po-tsu, a native of Nan Yang." In the *Chung-ching shih chuan kao* (仲景史傳考 Verification of Chang Chung-ching's Biography) written by Chang Tai-yen in the early years of the Republic of China (1911-) it says:

Having passed the second-degree officials' examination under the old system, Chang Chung-ching began the study of medicine under Chang Po-tsu of the same region. His knowledge and skills were said to be superior to those of his teacher.

Some authors state that Chang received a degree as doctor of literature in the reign of Ling Ti (A.D. 168). This has never been verified and would appear to be incorrect as this honor was probably not conferred at that time.

Disciples

There have been two pupils who were thought to have studied under Chang Chung-ching. The first disciple, Tu Tu, has not been proven a student conclusively as no record of his writings has been discovered. This, however, cannot rule out the possibility of his existence because many of the manuscripts of this period have been lost.

Reliable evidence does exist, however, relating to Chang's second follower Wei Fan. Chang Kuo said in his *I shuo* (醫說) (Medical Talks), "Wei Fan was good in medical therapy. He was taught medicine by Chang Chung-ching and became a learned physician." With this knowledge, Wei Fan was later able to contribute many valuable works on Chinese medicine. His theories are discussed in *Chein chin fang* (千金方 Precious Prescriptions), written by Sun Szu-mo (A.D. 590-682). In the *Hou han shu chang chung-ching chuan pu i* (後漢書張仲景傳補遺 Supplement to Chang Chi's Biography in the Later Han Historical Records) written by Lu Chiu-chih, the last sentence states, "His disciple Wei Fan was a well-informed physician." The omission of any mention of Tu Tu gives some credence to the theory that Chang had only one student although this cannot be regarded as conclusive.

Chang's Hall and Tomb

The medical sage's hall, which contains Chang's tomb, is situated to the west of Jen Chi bridge outside the Tung Kuo Gate in Nan Yang County, Honan Province. Following a visit to this area in 1933, Huang Chien wrote an interesting article entitled *Yeh nan yang i sheng chang chung-ching chi mu chi* (謁南陽醫聖張仲景祠墓記 Report on a Visit to the Medical Sage, Chang Chung-ching's Hall and Tomb in Nan Yang). He found the tomb located within the hall in front of which was an eight-foot stone tablet said to have been erected in 1657. (Some scholars feel that this stone is not authentic.) The area was built up and relics were gathered as a memorial and tribute to Chang's everlasting achievements. It has served as a place of veneration for subsequent pilgrimages.

Huang dates the inception of the shrine from a dream Feng Ying-ao had concerning Chang Chung-ching during an illness in 1628, the first year of the reign of Chung Chen of the Ming dynasty. Feng thereafter collected subscriptions until 1656, the thirteenth year of the reign of Shun Chih (Ming dynasty), thus making it possible to complete the structure in 1657. Huang felt that this date was accurate as there would have been many more stone tablets had the memorial been constructed in the Later Han dynasty.

Biography

An exact sequential biography of Chang has not been possible due to the lack of firm historical evidence from the Later Han dynasty. Some assumptions, therefore, will have to be made as a starting place for a possible chronology of his life. Sung Hsiang-yuan and Hung Kuan deduced that Chang was born in A.D. 147 and died in A.D. 219, whereas Cheng Pang-hsien placed his birth between the years A.D. 68 and A.D. 189 with the year of his death being uncertain.

Professor Chen Chau-yuen, a well-known Chinese medical practitioner in Hong Kong, subscribes to the following information. Chang Chung-ching was born in Nan Yang in A.D. 142

in the first year of the reign of Han An of the Later Han dynasty. He became acquainted with Ho Yu in A.D. 157 at the age of sixteen and four years later began to study medicine under the tutelage of Chang Po-tsu, both men being from the same region. Chang could have passed the second level officials' examination in A.D. 181 at the age of forty, but there is no evidence that he ever held any official position as a result. He became a friend of Wang Tsan, one of the famous "Seven Talents in the Chien-an Era" in A.D. 195 at the age of fifty-four. At that time he was practicing medicine in Ching Chou and had become adept in abdominal examination. It was reported that most of Chang's kindred died as a result of epidemics of a disease that spread throughout this area beginning in A.D. 196. As a result of this scourge, Chang was stimulated to study the cause, effects, and treatment of this pestilence preparatory to compiling the *Shang han tsa ping lun* (傷寒雜病論) in A.D. 200 at the age of fifty-nine. He completed the preface of the *Shang han lun* (傷寒 論) in A.D. 205 when he was sixty-four.

Chen also mentions the death of Hua To in A.D. 207, a contemporary and distinguished physician and surgeon who practiced in the region between Peng Cheng and Kuang Ling. Chen did not know whether or not these men were acquainted or if Hua was familiar with Chang's contributions to medicine. (Other comments in this respect have been noted above.) Chang died at the age of seventy-nine in A.D. 220, the first year of the reign of Yen Kang of the Wei dynasty (A.D. 220-265) in the period of the Three Kingdoms (Shu: A.D. 221-263; Wei: A.D. 220-265; and Wu: A.D. 222-280).

Part I

Shang han lun

by

Chang Chung – ching

Note: There is much disagreement among scholars as to the authorship of *Shang han lun*. The question is thoroughly discussed in Part II—A Study of the *Shang han lun*. However, we the publishers wish to emphasize here that we are of the opinion that the original, now lost, was written by Chang Chung-ching. It was later transcribed by Wang Su-ho who probably added to the original but did not alter its main body. The *Shang han lun* we know has thus come down to us from Wang Su-ho's copy.

1

Preface

Every time I read about Chin Yueh-jen's [also known as Pien
Chueh or Pien Ch'iao of Kuo—a state during the Warring States
Period] methods of diagnosis and his observations of the complexion of the Lord of Chi, I again admire his skills and talents.
I don't quite understand why scholars today do not pay more
attention to these formulas and techniques when treating their
elders, healing the poor, and maintaining their own health. They
do little but vie for fame and power and delight themselves with
improving their physical appearance while neglecting their spiritual
development. If one has no skin, how can there be any hair?
During a serious epidemic, victims of the disease become terri-
fied and do not know what to do. Under present circumstances
they must submit themselves to the care of witch doctors or
depend upon divine providence in the hope of prolonging their
lives. Alas! It is a foolish world that indulges itself in the acquisi-
tion of fame and wealth and regards life so lightly. Is this the true
meaning of glory and power? People who compete for superficial
success without caring for the essentials, who are indifferent to
bodily care and indulge only in material gain, are as much in
danger as though walking on an icy bridge abutting a valley.
One who fails to learn how to love both others and oneself is not
unlike a homeless, wandering spirit seeking transitory worldly
pleasures.

During the first ten years of the Chien-an era (A.D. 196)
of the Later Han dynasty, two-thirds of my relatives (more than
two hundred) succumbed to disease, seven-tenths of which

2

(deaths) were due to an epidemic fever. For this reason and in consideration of all those lost and not saved in the past, I decided to seek diligently ancient instrutions and try to adopt for use various well-known formulas. I then studied the *Su wen* (Simple Questions in the Yellow Emperor's Classic of Internal Medicine in nine volumes called *Ling shu*, Mystical Gate, or Pivot of Life), *Nan ching* (The Eighty-one Perplexities also called the Classic of Medical Perplexities or the Difficult Classic), and *Yin yang ta lun* (The Great Treatise of Yin and Yang) herb book, and pulse books. (See Appendices 1-5 for more information on these books.)

I now have written the book *Shang han tsa ping lun* (The Classic of Febrile and Miscellaneous Diseases). Although it does not include all therapies, the book tells of the cause and origin of the majority of diseases. The reader will gain much medical knowledge if he makes a thorough study of my compilation.

Heaven with the five elements governs all creatures. Man with his five constant virtues possesses the five organs. There are many yet undiscovered mysteries and unknown changes in the interactions of the meridians, vessels, points, and yin and yang. Only a man with inordinate ability and profound knowledge can understand medical truths and mechanisms of illness. Many famous medical practitioners lived in ancient times including Shen Nung, Huang Ti (the Yellow Emperor), Chi Po, Po Kao, Lei Kung, Shao Shu, and Chung Wen. In later ages Chang Sang and Pien Chueh (Pien Ch'iao or Chin Yueh-jen) were fine physicians and finally in the Han dynasty were Officer Yang Ching and Chang Kung (Ts'ang Kung, Ch'un Yu-i, or Shun Yu-i), but thereafter there have been none.

Physicians today do not thoroughly study the medical classics before they begin to practice but merely follow their predecessors with no attempt to improve age-old form words (remedies). Herb teas are administered after only a brief conversation with the patient. They take the front (superficial, external, or *fu*) pulse but not the rear (deep, internal, or *ch'en*); check the hands but not the feet; and do not make a diagnosis of the complete upper, middle, and lower parts of the body. How can a pulse rate alone and careless observation tell about all the confirmations and diseases? It is difficult to restore life to a patient near death. This is comparable to observing the sky through a tube that shows

3

only a very small portion of the whole.

Confucius said, "A superior man is born with talent but even he like an ordinary man needs to work hard in order to obtain a wide range of learning." Having studied medicine for a long period, I wish to record this aphorism in closing as an encouragement to all students.

Chapter One
Greater Yang Disease

1. 太陽之爲病，脈浮，頭項強痛，而惡寒。

   The primary symptoms of greater yang diseases are floating pulse, headache, stiffness of the neck, and severe chills. These are called surface symptoms.

2. 太陽病，發熱汗出，惡風，脈緩者，名爲中風。

   In greater yang disease, perspiration due to fever, mild chills (or anemophobia[1]) and a slow pulse are termed *chung feng*, a mild form of greater yang disease.

3. 太陽病，或已發熱，或未發熱，必惡寒，體痛，嘔逆，脈陰陽俱緊者，名曰傷寒。

   A more severe type of greater yang disease, with or without fever, is called *shang han* and is associated with severe chills, generalized aching, vomiting, hiccoughs, and a tense pulse when palpated deeply as well as superficially.

4. 太陽中風，脈陽浮而陰弱，嗇嗇惡寒，淅淅惡風，翕翕發熱，鼻鳴，乾嘔者，桂枝湯主之。

   The *chung feng* form of greater yang disease accompanied by

5

a floating pulse (superficial palpation) or weak pulse (deep palpation), mild or severe chills, persistent fever, nasal irritation and congestion, and nausea should be treated primarily with *Kuei-chih-tang* (Cinnamon Combination).

5. 太陽病，頭痛發熱，汗出惡風者，桂枝湯主之。
Kuei-chih-tang (Cinnamon Combination) should be given [to patients with] greater yang disease who have headaches, fever, perspiration, and mild chills (anemophobia).

6. 太陽病，項背強几几，反汗出，惡風者，桂枝加葛根湯主之。
Greater yang disease with symptoms of stiffness in the neck and back [muscles are extended], perspiration, and mild chills (anemophobia) should be treated mainly with *Kuei-chih-chia-ko-ken-tang* (Cinnamon and Pueraria Combination).

7. 太陽病，下之後，其氣上衝者，可與桂枝湯。
Kuei-chih-tang (Cinnamon Combination) is given [for cases of] greater yang disease that have been treated with the purgation method [but have upward] congestion [from the chest to the pharynx].

8. 太陽病，三日，已發汗，若吐，若下，若溫針，仍不解者，此為壞病。
If there is no response after the first three days to treatment with the sweating, vomiting, and purgation methods or acupuncture with [moxibustion] in greater yang diseases, the condition has been treated improperly.

9. 太陽病，發汗，遂漏不止，其人惡風，小便難，四肢微急，難以屈伸者，桂枝加附子湯主之。
Greater yang disease with continuous perspiration, mild chills (anemophobia), difficulty in urination, and muscle spasms of the limbs which make it difficult to flex and extend the arms and legs should be treated essentially with *Kuei-chih-chia-fu-tzu-tang* (Cinnamon, Aconite, and Jujube Combination).

10. 太陽病下之後，脈促胸滿者，桂枝去芍藥湯主之。若微惡寒者，

6

桂枝去芍藥加附子湯主之 。

If there is a fast pulse and fullness of the chest after treatment of greater yang disease with the purgation method, therapy with *Kuei-chih-chu-shao-yao-tang* (Cinnamon Minus Paeonia Combination) is suggested. In case the disease is accompanied by a somewhat severe chill [after perspiring], the condition should be treated chiefly with *Kuei-chih-chu-shao-yao-chia-fu-tzu-tang* (Cinnamon, Ginger, and Aconite Combination).

11. 太陽病，得之八九日，如瘧狀，發熱惡寒，熱多寒少，其人不嘔，清便欲自可，一日二三度發，以其不能得少汗出，身必癢，宜桂枝麻黃各半湯 。

Kuei-chih-ma-huang-ko-pan-tang (Cinnamon and *Ma-huang* Combination) is recommended for greater yang disease that has been present for eight to nine days with muscular spasms along with malaria-like symptoms— [alternating] fever and severe chills (the fever being of longer duration than the chills) without vomiting and with normal bowel function— [as well as for cases with] two or three [mild] daily relapses [of malaria-like symptoms] without perspiration but with pruritus. (See Appendix 6 for further information.)

12. 太陽病，初服桂枝湯，反煩不解者，先刺風池風府，卻與桂枝湯則愈 。

If after the first administration of *Kuei-chih-tang* (Cinnamon Combination) for greater yang disease there is continued distress instead of recovery, acupuncture should be performed at points *feng chih* (G20) and *feng fu* (GV16) [in order to disperse *ch'i*]. Then *Kuei-chih-tang* is given again to effect a cure.

13. 服桂枝湯，大汗出，脈洪大者，與桂枝湯，如前法。若形如瘧，一日再發者，汗出必解，宜桂枝二麻黃一湯 。

In the presence of continued profuse sweating and a large pulse [without thirst] after one administration of *Kuei-chih-tang* (Cinnamon Combination), a second dose should be given as recommended in the preceding paragraph. If [improvement is not complete and] there are [mild], daily, recurring malaria-like symptoms [but no perspiration], recovery will be delayed until perspiration occurs. *Kuei-chih-erh-ma-huang-i-tang (Ma-huang* and Double Cinnamon Combination) is recommended under these circumstances.

14. 服桂枝湯，大汗出後，大煩渴不解，脈洪大者，白虎加人參湯主之。

If severe perspiration, marked distress, prolonged thirst, and a large pulse persist after taking *Kuei-chih-tang* (Cinnamon Combination), *Pai-hu-chia-jen-sheng-tang* (Ginseng and Gypsum Combination) should be taken.

15. 太陽病，發熱惡寒，熱多寒少，脈微弱者，不可發大汗，宜桂枝二越婢一湯。

Kuei-chih-erh-yueh-pei-i-tang (Cinnamon, *Ma-huang,* and Gypsum Combination) is recommended instead of the sweating method in greater yang disease [characterized] by sustained fever of a longer duration than the severe chills with which it alternates. However, an initiation of profuse sweating should be avoided in the presence of a minute and weak pulse [due to the lack of yang].

16. 服桂枝湯，復下之，仍頭項強痛，翕翕發熱，無汗，心下滿微痛，小便不利者，桂枝去桂加茯苓白朮湯主之。

[Those cases treated with] *Kuei-chih-tang* (Cinnamon Combination) and the purgation method in which there are still headaches, stiffness of the neck, persistent fever without perspiration, fullness beneath the heart with mild aching, and dysuria, should be given *Kuei-chih-chu-kuei-chia-fu-ling-pai-chu-tang* (Hoelen, Atractylodes, and Paeonia Combination).

17. 傷寒，脈浮，自汗出，小便數，心煩，微惡寒，脚攣急．反與桂枝湯。得之便厥，咽中乾，煩躁、吐逆者，作甘草乾薑湯，與之。若厥愈，足溫者，更作芍藥甘草湯，與之。若胃氣不和，讝語者，少與調胃承氣湯。若重發汗，復加燒針，得之者，四逆湯主之。

[Cases of the] *shang han* [condition] that exhibit a floating pulse, spontaneous perspiration, polyuria, distress, mild chills, and foot spasms should not be treated with *Kuei-chih-tang* (Cinnamon Combination) as it would cause more severe chills in the limbs, dryness of the pharynx, continued distress, and vomiting. These patients require *Kan-tsao-kan-chiang-tang* (Licorice and Ginger Combination). [The yang has been restored] if the chills disappear and the feet regain their warmth. Administration of *Shao-yao-kan-tsao-tang* (Paeonia and Licorice Combination) shall then follow [to restore the yin]. A small portion of *Tiao-wei-cheng-chi-tang* (Rhubarb and Mirabilitum Combination) is given to patients with stomach disorders and delirium. Cases with recurrent perspiration aggravated by the use of moxibustion should be treated mainly with *Szu-ni-tang* (Aconite, Ginger, and Licorice Combination).

18. 太陽病．項背強几几，無汗惡風，葛根湯主之。

Greater yang disease in which there is a sensation of stiffness and heaviness in the neck and back, mild chills (anemophobia), but no perspiration, should be given *Ko-ken-tang* (Pueraria Combination).

19. 太陽與陽明合病者，必自下利，葛根湯主之。

Ko-ken-tang (Pueraria Combination) is given to patients experiencing diarrhea as a complication of greater and sunlight yang diseases.

20. 太陽與陽明合病，不下利，但嘔者，葛根加半夏湯主之。

Ko-ken-chia-pan-hsia-tang (Pueraria and Pinellia Combination) is given to patients with vomiting, but without diarrhea, as a complication of greater and sunlight yang diseases.

21. 太陽病，桂枝證，醫反下之，利遂不止，喘而汗出者，葛根黃連黃芩甘草湯主之。

Ko-ken-huang-lien-huang-chin-kan-tsao-tang (L. S. C. and Pueraria Combination) is indicated for the Cinnamon confirmation of greater yang disease. This is when continuous diarrhea, gasping, and perspiration occur following an adverse treatment with the purgation method.

22. 太陽病，頭痛發熱，身疼腰痛，骨節疼痛，惡風，無汗而喘者，麻黃湯主之。

Greater yang disease with [the symptoms] of headache, fever, generalized discomfort, low back pain, aching of the joints, mild chills (anemophobia), and gasping, but no per-spiration, is treated with *Ma-huang-tang* (*Ma-huang* Combination).

23. 太陽中風，脈浮緊，發熱惡寒，身疼痛，不汗出而煩躁者，大青龍湯主之。若脈微弱，汗出惡風者，不可服之。服之則厥逆，筋惕肉瞤。

The *chung feng* [condition] of greater yang disease [is characterized by] a floating, tense pulse; alternating fever and severe chills; generalized aching; distress; and the absence of perspiration. This condition should be treated mainly with *Ta-ching-lung-tang* (Major Blue Dragon Combination). For patients with a feeble, weak pulse; perspiration; and mild chills (anemophobia), this herb formula is contraindicated as it may cause chills of the distal limbs and muscular spasms.

24. 傷寒，脈浮緩，身不疼，但重，乍有輕時，大青龍湯主之。

Ta-ching-lung-tang (Major Blue Dragon Combination) is given for *shang han* in which there is a floating and slow pulse and a sensation of heaviness with occasional weakness [rather than] generalized body aches.

25. 傷寒表不解，心下有水氣，乾嘔發熱而欬，或渴，或利，或噎，或小便不利，小腹滿，或喘者，小青龍湯主之。

Hsiao-ching-lung-tang (Minor Blue Dragon Combination) is indicated for *shang han* [conditions] when the surface symptoms—water (fluid) beneath the heart, retching, fever, cough, thirst, diarrhea, hiccoughs, dysuria, fullness of the lower abdomen, and gasping—are not relieved.

26. 傷寒，心下有水氣，欬有微喘，發熱不渴，小青龍湯主之。

Shang han [conditions] with water (fluid) beneath the heart resulting in a cough, mild gasping, and fever without thirst should be treated primarily with *Hsiao-ching-lung-tang* (Minor Blue Dragon Combination).

27. 太陽病，外證未解，脈浮弱者，當以汗解，宜桂枝湯。

When the outside confirmation of greater yang disease is not relieved by the sweating method [as evidenced by] a floating and weak pulse, *Kuei-chih-tang* (Cinnamon Combination) may be given.

28. 太陽病下之，微喘者，表未解故也，桂枝加厚朴杏子湯主之。

Mild gasping indicates that the surface symptoms of greater yang disease have not been corrected even after using the purgation method. This [condition] should be treated primarily with *Kuei-chih-chia-hou-pu-hsing-jen-tang* (M. A. and Cinnamon Combination).

29. 太陽病，外證未解，不可下也，欲解外者，宜桂枝湯。

When the surface confirmation [of *Kuei-chih-tang*] of greater yang disease is not relieved, *Kuei-chih-tang* (Cinnamon Combination) is recommended rather than the purgation method.

30. 太陽病，脈浮緊，無汗發熱身疼痛，八九日不解，表證仍在，其人發煩目瞑，劇者必衄，麻黄湯主之。

When greater yang disease with a floating and tense pulse, fever and generalized aching, but no perspiration, has not improved in eight or nine days, it indicates that there is still a surface confirmation. [If] the patient also suffers from anxiety and dizziness and in severe cases epistaxis, *Ma-huang-tang* (*Ma-huang* Combination) is given.

31. 二陽併病，太陽初得病時，發其汗，汗先出不徹，因轉屬陽明，續自微汗出，不惡寒，如此可以小發汗。設面色緣緣正赤者，陽氣拂鬱，不得越，其人短氣，但坐，更發汗則愈。

If treatment of the primary stage of greater yang disease with the sweating method does not result in thorough perspiring as desired, the condition shifts to the sunlight yang category, [a complication of greater yang and sunlight yang diseases]. If spontaneous perspiration continues without severe chills, a mild sweating method may be used. In case the patient has an intensely ruddy complexion—evidence that the yang *ch'i* (evil *ch'i*) is suppressed and not dispersed—rapid respiration, and [an agonized condition in which he] cannot lie down, only sit up, he can be cured by an additional sweating treatment.

32. 傷寒，脈浮緊，不發汗，因致衄者，麻黄湯主之。

The *shang han* [condition] associated with a floating and tense pulse, no perspiration, and a nosebleed should be treated primarily with *Ma-huang-tang* (*Ma-huang* Combination).

11

33. 發汗後，身疼痛，脈沈遲者，桂枝加芍藥生薑各一兩人參三兩新加湯主之。

[The patient] with generalized aching and a sinking and slow pulse should be treated, after inducing perspiration, mainly with *Hsin-chia-tang* [Cinnamon Combination to which has been added one *liang* (31.25 grams) each of paeonia and ginger and three *liang* (93.75 grams) of ginseng].

34. 發汗後，喘家，不可更行桂枝湯。汗出喘，無大熱者，可與麻黄杏仁甘草石膏湯。

[The patient] who gasps after perspiring should not be given additional *Kuei-chih-tang* (Cinnamon Combination). Those without a severe fever [who are subject to] gasping after perspiring may be given *Ma-hsing-kan-shih-tang* (Apricot Seed and *Ma-huang* Combination).

35. 發汗過多，其人叉手自冒心，心下悸，欲得按者，桂枝甘草湯主之。

Kuei-chih-kan-tsao-tang (Cinnamon and Licorice Combination) is given [to patients] with profuse perspiration and rapid heart palpitations, [the latter causing] the patient to cross his hands over his heart and press firmly.

36. 發汗後，其人臍下悸者，欲作奔豚，茯苓桂枝甘草大棗湯主之。

[The patient] with palpitation beneath the umbilicus and distention beneath the heart, after inducing sweating, should be treated mainly with *Fu-ling-kuei-chih-kan-tsao-ta-tsao-tang* (C. L. J. and Hoelen Combination).

37. 發汗後，腹脹滿者，厚朴生薑半夏甘草人參湯主之。

Hou-pu-sheng-chiang-pan-hsia-kan-tsao-jen-sheng-tang (Magnolia Five Combination) should be given to [patients] with abdominal distention after sweating has been induced.

38. 傷寒，若吐若下後，心下逆滿，氣上衝胸，起則頭眩，脈沈緊，發汗則動經，身為振振搖者，茯苓桂枝白朮甘草湯主之。

[For] *shang han* [conditions] after the vomiting and purgation methods have been used, [if there is still] a fullness beneath the heart, chest distention, dizziness when standing up, a skinking and tight pulse, and if there has been an injury to the yang meridian manifested by perspiration and a generalized unsteadiness, *Fu-ling-kuei-chih-pai-chu-kan-tsao-tang* (Hoelen, Licorice, and Atractylodes Combination) is recommended.

39. 發汗，病不解，反惡寒者，芍藥甘草附子湯主之。

If the above symptoms are not relieved [and the patient] continues to have chills after perspiring, *Shao-yao-kan-tsao-fu-tzu-tang* (Paeonia, Licorice, and Aconite Combination) is prescribed.

40. 發汗若下之，病仍不解，煩躁者，茯苓四逆湯主之。

[If the patient] does not improve after perspiring or the use of the purgation method and experiences distress and anxiety, he should be treated primarily with *Fu-ling-szu-ni-tang* (Hoelen, Licorice, Aconite, and Ginseng Combination).

41. 發汗後惡寒者，虛故也，不惡寒，但熱者，實也，當和胃氣，與調胃承氣湯。

[The patient] who has severe chills after perspiring is of the weak type; (patients) with fever but no severe chills [following perspiring] are of the strong type. The stomach reaction of the strong type should be harmonized by administering *Tiao-wei-cheng-chi-tang* (Rhubarb and Mirabilitum Combination).

42. 太陽病，發汗後，大汗出，胃中乾，煩躁不得眠，欲得飲水者，少少與飲之，令胃氣和則愈。若脈浮，小便不利，微熱，消渴者，五苓散主之。

A little water will settle the stomach and cure patients with greater yang disease that manifests dryness in the stomach after profuse perspiration induced by a sweating treatment, insomnia caused by anxiety and irritability, and a desire to drink water. *Wu-ling-san* (Hoelen Five Herb Formula) is preferred for those cases with a floating pulse, dysuria, mild fever, and [diabetic-like] thirst.

13

43. 發汗巳，脈浮數，煩渴者，五苓散主之。

Wu-ling-san (Hoelen Five Herb Formula) is recommended [for patients] with a floating and rapid pulse, distress, and thirst after perspiring.

44. 傷寒汗出而渴者，五苓散主之。不渴者，茯苓甘草湯主之。

Wu-ling-san (Hoelen Five Herb Formula) is given for shang han (condition) with perspiration and thirst. [Patients who are] perspiring but not thirsty should be given Fu-ling-kan-tsao-tang (Hoelen and Licorice Combination).

45. 中風，發熱六七日，不解而煩，渴欲飲水，水入口吐者，五苓散主之。

Wu-ling-san (Hoelen Five Herb Formula) should be given for chung feng [conditions] exhibiting a persistent, unrelieved fever over a period of six to seven days, along with symptoms of anxiety, intense thirst, and vomiting after ingestion of fluids.

46. 發汗吐下後，虛煩不得眠，若劇者，必反覆顛倒，心中懊憹，梔子豉湯主之。若少氣者，梔子甘草豉湯主之。若嘔者，梔子生薑豉湯主之。

Patients who after sweating, vomiting, and purgation treatments experience weakness, anxiety, and insomnia, as well as irritability and restlessness in the more serious cases, should take Chih-tzu-shih-tang (Gardenia and Soja Combination). Patients with short [rapid] breathing should primarily take Chih-tzu-kan-tsao-shih-tang (Gardenia, Licorice, and Soja Combination), while Chih-tzu-sheng-chiang-shih-tang (Gardenia, Ginger, and Soja Combination) should be given in cases with vomiting.

47. 發汗若下之，而煩熱胸中窒者，梔子豉湯主之。

Chih-tzu-shih-tang (Gardenia and Soja Combination) is indicated for patients who after undergoing the sweating treatment followed by a purgation treatment experience stagnancy in the chest due to anxiety and fever.

48. 傷寒五六日，大下之後，身熱不去，心中結痛者，未欲解也，梔子豉湯主之。

If the *shang han* [condition] persists for five to six days following strong purgation [with the disease shifting from the greater to the lesser yang stage], the lingering fever and thoracic stagnancy and aching may be relieved by *Chih-tzu-shih-tang* (Gardenia and Soja Combination).

49. 傷寒下後，心煩腹滿，臥起不安者，梔子厚朴湯主之。

Shang han [conditions] treated by the purgation method that [still exhibit continued] distress, a sensation of fullness of the stomach, and restlessness should be treated with *Chih-tzu-hou-pu-tang* (Gardenia and Magnolia Combination).

50. 傷寒，醫以丸藥，大下之，身熱不去，微煩者，梔子乾薑湯主之。

Patients with *shang han* [conditions] that have been purged excessively with pillular herbs by the physician but who continue to have generalized fever and slight distress due to weakness should take *Chih-tzu-kan-chiang-tang* (Gardenia and Ginger Combination).

51. 下之後，發汗，晝日煩躁，不得眠，夜而安靜，不嘔，不渴，無表證，脈沈微，身無大熱者，乾薑附子湯主之。

A patient treated with the purgation method [followed by] the sweating method may [continue to] experience anxiety and difficulty in sleeping during the day [due to the yang being on the verge of exhaustion] but not at night [due to a preponderance of yin]. This condition is not accompanied by vomiting [absence of lesser yang confirmation], and thirst [lack of sunlight yang disease confirmation]. The patient also will have a surface confirmation of headaches, severe chills, and a generalized fever with a sinking (inside) and weak (absent yang) pulse. In this case, *Kan-chiang-fu-tzu-tang* (Ginger and Aconite Combination) is indicated [to warm the body and restore yang].

52. 太陽病、發汗、汗出不解、其人仍發熱，心下悸，頭眩，身瞤動，振振欲擗者，玄武湯主之。

If the patient continues to have a fever, rapid heart palpitation, vertigo, trembling, and a tendency to collapse after perspiring which has been induced by the sweating method, he still has a greater yang disease and should be treated mainly with *Hsuan-wu-tang* (Vitality Combination) [but the disease has entered the lesser yin confirmation].

53. 傷寒，醫下之，續得下利，清穀不止，身疼痛者，急當救裏，後身疼痛，清便自調者，急當救表，救裏宜四逆湯，救表宜桂枝湯。

For *shang han* [conditions already] treated by a physician with the purgation method [which still exhibit both] continued diarrhea containing undigested food, and generalized aching, the inside of the body should be nourished at once with a warm drug like *Szu-ni-tang* (Ginger, Licorice, and Aconite Combination) to strengthen the weak gastrointestinal function. If the generalized aching persists [after treatment] but the stool has become normal, then the patient should be treated at once for the surfacial confirmation with *Kuei-chih-tang* (Cinnamon Combination).

54. 傷寒五六日，往來寒熱，胸脇苦滿，默默不欲飲食，心煩喜嘔，或胸中煩而不嘔，或渴，或腹中痛，或脇下痞鞕，或心下悸，小便不利，或不渴，身有微熱，或欬者，小柴胡湯主之。

If the *shang han* [condition] persists for five to six days with alternating chills and fever, distress and fullness in the chest and ribs, silence with loss of appetite, disturbances in the heart with a tendency to vomit or disturbances in the chest without vomiting, thirst, abdominal aching, obstruction and stiffness beneath the ribs; or palpitations beneath the heart, dysuria, adypsia, mild generalized fever, or cough, *Hsiao-chai-hu-tang* (Minor Bupleurum Combination) is indicated.

55. 傷寒四五日，身熱惡風，頸項強，脇下滿，手足溫而渴者，小柴胡湯主之。

For *shang han* [conditions that have persisted] for four to five days with somatic fever, severe chills, stiffness of the neck, fullness beneath the ribs, warm limbs, and thirst, *Hsiao-chai-hu-tang* (Minor Bupleurum Combination) is indicated.

56. 傷寒，陽脈濇，陰脈弦，法當腹中急痛，先與小建中湯，不差者，
小柴胡湯主之。

[Patients with a] *shang han* condition with an obstructed,
rough pulse on superficial palpation and a tense pulse on
deep touch will have an acute abdominal ache and should
first take *Hsiao-chien-chung-tang* (Minor Cinnamon and
Paeonia Combination). If recovery is not complete, *Hsiao-
chai-hu-tang* (Minor Bupleurum Combination) should be
taken.

57. 傷寒二三日，心中悸而煩者，小建中湯主之。

Shang han [conditions continuing] for two or three days
with rapid heart palpitation and distress [which cannot be
treated with the sweating method due to a deficiency of
yang] should be treated primarily with *Hsiao-chien-chung-
tang* (Minor Cinnamon and Paeonia Combination).

58. 太陽病，十餘日，反二三下之，後四五日，柴胡證仍在者，先
與小柴胡湯。嘔不止，心下急，鬱鬱微煩者，為未解也，與大
柴胡湯，下之則愈。

Sometimes greater yang disease persists for more than ten
days and moves slowly into the lesser yang stage. If it has
been mistakenly treated with two or three purgations [under
the assumption that the disease has shifted to the sunlight
yang stage] and four or five days later it still exhibits *Chai-
hu-tang* confirmation, it should now be treated with *Hsiao-
chai-hu-tang* (Minor Bupleurum Combination). In cases of
severe vomiting [after taking this combination], plus unrelieved stagnancy beneath the heart and distress in the chest,
treatment with *Ta-chai-hu-tang* (Major Bupleurum Combination) may result in recovery after an episode of diarrhea.

59. 傷寒十三日不解，胸脇滿而嘔，日晡所發潮熱，已而微利，先
宜服小柴胡湯以解外，後以柴胡加芒硝湯主之。

If the *shang han* condition has persisted for about thirteen
days with fullness between the chest and ribs, vomiting
[lesser yang and *Chai-hu-tang* (Bupleurum Combination) con-
firmation], tide fever at sunset [sunlight yang and *Ch'eng-
chi-tang* (Rhubarb Combination) confirmation] and mild
diarrhea, *Hsiao-chai-hu-tang* (Minor Bupleurum Combination)

17

is recommended to relieve the surface symptoms followed by *Chai-hu-chia-mang-hsiao-tang* (Bupleurum and Mirabilitum Combination). [These herbal formulas will treat both lesser and sunlight yang confirmations.]

60. 太陽病不解，熱結膀胱，其人如狂，血自下。其外不解者，尚未可攻。當先解其外，外解已，但小腹急結者，乃可攻之，宜桃核承氣湯。

An unrelieved greater yang disease that exhibits a feverish lower warmer (the area between the stomach and the bladder) will result in extravasated blood which in turn will cause delirium in the patient. This condition may be helped by eliminating the extravasated blood in a bloody stool. However, if the surface symptoms do not improve with or without a bloody stool, purgative herbs should not further be administered. The surface symptoms should be relieved first and when this is done, the acute lower abdominal pain may be dispersed with *Tao-ho-cheng-chi-tang* (Persica and Rhubarb Combination).

61. 傷寒八九日，下之，胸滿煩驚，小便不利，讝語，一身盡重，不可轉側者，柴胡加龍骨牡蠣湯主之。

[The patient still suffering from] a *shang han* [condition] for eight or nine days after treatment with the purgation method [with a feeling of] fullness in the chest, anxiety and nervousness, dysuria, delirium, heaviness of body, and difficulty in turning should be treated mainly with *Chai-hu-chia-lung-ku-mu-li-tang* (Bupleurum and Dragon Bone Combination).

62. 傷寒，脈浮，醫以火迫劫之，必驚狂，臥起不安者，桂枝去芍藥加蜀漆牡蠣龍骨救逆湯主之。

A *shang han* [condition] with a floating pulse already treated with a burnt needle (acupuncture and moxibustion) where the patient continues to exhibit nervousness, fear, insomnia, and emotional instability should be treated with *Kuei-chih-chu-shao-yao-chia-shu-chi-lung-ku-mu-li-chiu-ni-tang* (Cinnamon, Dichroa, Oyster Shell and Dragon Bone Combination).

63. 太陽病，以火熏之，不得汗，其人必躁，必清血，名為火邪。

The term "harmful heat" is applied to [cases of] greater yang disease which have failed to perspire after a fire-fumigation treatment, and always end in irritability and bloody stools [because the heat has attacked the inside]. These patients will also show a tendency towards anxiety which can be cured by purgation.

64. 燒針令其汗，針處被寒，核起而赤者，必發奔豚，灸其核上各一壯，與桂枝加桂湯。

If greater yang disease has been treated with the burnt needle method to render perspiration and the site of insertion has been invaded by chills and a red, swollen nucleus has developed thereon, it can be cured by applying one single unit of moxa on the site followed by *Kuei-chih-chia-kuei-tang*(Cinnamon, Licorice, and Ginger Combination).

65. 火逆，下之，因燒針，煩躁者，桂枝甘草龍骨牡蠣湯主之。

Patients with distress as a result of harmful heat due to the previous use of acupuncture with moxibustion or the use of the purgation method should be given *Kuei-chih-kan-tsao-lung-ku-mu-li-tang* (Cinnamon, Licorice, Oyster Shell, and Dragon Bone Combination).

66. 太陽病，十餘日，心下溫溫欲吐，而胸中痛，大便反溏，腹微滿，鬱鬱微煩，先此時，自極吐下者，與調胃承氣湯。

Greater yang disease which persists for more than ten days with heart distress, gagging, aching in the chest, loose stools (the condition has now entered into the sunlight yang category), mild abdominal distention, depression, and mild anxiety, and, prior to these symptoms, severe vomiting and diarrhea [occurred spontaneously], should be treated with *Tiao-wei-cheng-chi-tang* (Rhubarb and Mirabilitum Combination).

67. 太陽病，六七日，表證仍在，脈微而沈，反不結胸，其人發狂者，以熱在下焦，小腹當鞕滿。小便自利者，下血乃愈，抵當湯主之。

Greater yang disease that has lasted six or seven days, but which has not yet become a lesser yang condition, that exhibits residual surface symptoms, a feeble (superficial palpation) and sinking pulse (deep palpation), an absence of stagnancy in the chest, delirium [due to] fever in the lower

19

warmer, hardness and fullness of the lower abdomen, and polyuria [associated with blood stagnation] may be cured by a discharge of blood and should be given *Ti-tang-tang* (Rhubarb and Leech Combination).

68. 太陽病，身黄，脈沈結，小腹鞭，小便自利，其人如狂者，抵當湯主之。

Greater yang disease that exhibits a yellowish skin, sinking and knotted pulse, hardness of the lower abdomen, polyuria, and a manic state should be treated primarily with *Ti-tang-tang* (Rhubarb and Leech Combination).

69. 傷寒有熱，小腹滿，應小便不利。今反利者，當下之，宜抵當丸。

Shang han [conditions] of fever and fullness in the lower stomach where there is dysuria instead of polyuria should be purged and treated with *Ti-tang-wan* (Rhubarb and Leech Formula).

70. 結胸者，項亦强，如柔痙狀，下之則和，宜大陷胸丸。

[A patient with distention and] hardness in the chest, plus stiffness and mild spasms of the neck, should be treated with the purgation method and given *Ta-hsien-hsiung-wan* (Major Rhubarb and Mirabilitum Formula).

71. 太陽病，脈浮而動數，頭痛發熱，微盜汗出，而反惡寒者，表未解也，醫反下之，動數變遲，膈内拒痛，短氣躁煩，心中懊憹，陽氣内陷，心下因鞭，則爲結胸。大陷胸湯主之。若不結胸，但頭汗出，餘處無汗，劑頸而還，小便不利，身心發黄。

If the surface symptoms of greater yang disease—a floating and fast pulse, headache, fever, mild night sweats, and severe chills—are not relieved and the physician [initiates] treatment with the purgation method, these surface symptoms will internalize. As a result there will be a slowing of the pulse, aching of the chest, rapid respiration, severe anxiety due to yang *ch'i* internalizing and becoming harmful, and distress in the heart accompanied by hardness due to stagnancy. Treatment with *Ta-hsien-hsiung-tang* (Rhubarb and *Kan-sui* Combination) is then indicated. Cases without stagnancy in the chest but with perspiration in the head area

20

but not on the rest of the body, and with difficult urination, will eventually result in a yellowing of the skin (jaundice) and eyes.

72. 傷寒六七日，結胸熱實，脈沈而緊，心下痛，按之石鞭者，大陷胸湯主之。

Shang han [conditions] lasting six or seven days with stagnancy in the chest, a "heat-firm" confirmation [indicating that the disease has invaded the body], a sinking and tense pulse, and aching beneath the heart where it feels as hard as a stone, should be treated primarily with *Ta-hsien-hsiung-tang* (Rhubarb and *Kan-sui* Combination).

73. 傷寒十餘日，熱結在裏，復往來寒熱者，與大柴胡湯，但結胸無大熱，但頭微汗出者，大陷胸湯主之。

For *shang han* [conditions] which persist for longer than ten days and exhibit an accumulation of heat within the body, together with alternating chills and fever, [this is the fever type of lesser yang disease] *Ta-chai-hu-tang* (Major Bupleurum Combination) should be given. When there is [water] stagnancy in the chest without surface fever [or alternating chills and fever] and only mild perspiration confined to the head [due to flushing up of water toxin], *Ta-hsien-hsiung-tang* (Rhubarb and *Kan-sui* Combination) should be given.

74. 太陽病，重發汗而復下之，不大便五六日，舌上燥而渴，日晡所小有潮熱，從心下至小腹，鞭滿而痛，不可近者，大陷胸湯主之。

If greater yang disease has been treated twice by the sweating method and once by the purgation method [resulting in loss of body fluids for four to five days] and if there is no bowel movement for an additional five to six days, [the patient's condition has advanced to the sunlight yang stage of the disease]. His symptoms of dryness of the tongue, thirst, mild tide fever at the end of the day, and hardness with fullness and aching that hurts violently upon the slightest touch from beneath the heart to the lower abdomen should be treated mainly with *Ta-hsien-hsiung-tang* (Rhubarb and *Kan-sui* Combination).

75. 小結胸者，正在心下，按之則痛，脈浮滑者，小陷胸湯主之。

Minor stagnancy in the chest localized beneath the heart which results in pain on palpation [and is accompanied by] a floating and smooth pulse should be given *Hsiao-hsien-hsiung-tang* (Minor Trichosanthes Combination).

76. 病在陽，應以汗解之。反以冷水潠之，若灌之，其熱被劫不得去，彌更益煩，肉上粟起。意欲飲水，反小渴者，服文蛤散。若不差者，與五苓散。若寒實結胸，無熱證者，與三物小白散。

Illness (fever, etc.) localized in the temporal area of the head should be treated with the sweating method (Cinnamon or *Ma-huang* Combination). Water applied to [the temples] represses the heat and it cannot be dispersed. This results in severe anxiety, goose flesh (cutis anserina), and thirst which ceases immediately upon drinking. This condition calls for *Wen-ke-san* (Meretrix Formula); if a cure is not achieved, *Wu-ling-san* (Hoelen Five Herb Formula) is indicated. In cases with no heat confirmation but with cold inside which has accumulated in the chest, *San-wu-hsiao-pai-san* (Platycondon and Croton Formula) is given.

77. 婦人中風七八日，續得寒熱，發作有時，經水適斷者，其血必結，故使如瘧狀，發作有時，小柴胡湯主之。

Women with *chung feng* [conditions] lasting seven to eight days, lingering chills and fever occurring at regular intervals (malaria-like symptoms), and amenorrhea and stagnancy of the blood should be treated primarily with *Hsiao-chai-hu-tang* (Minor Bupleurum Combination).[2]

78. 傷寒六七日，發熱微惡寒，支節煩疼，微嘔，心下支結，外證未去者，柴胡桂枝湯主之。

Shang han [conditions] lasting six or seven days with fever, mild [inside] chills, persisting aching in the limbs [surface confirmation], mild vomiting, and distention beneath the heart require *Chai-hu-kuei-chih-tang* (Bupleurum and Cinnamon Combination). These symptoms signify that an outside confirmation still exists in the temporal areas.

79. 傷寒五六日，已發汗，而復下之，胸脇滿微結，小便不利，渴而不嘔，但頭汗出，往來寒熱，心煩者，柴胡桂枝乾薑湯主之。

Shang han [conditions] lasting five to six days that have been treated first with the sweating method and then the purgation method but exhibit [continued] fullness and congestion in the chest, dysuria, thirst without vomiting, perspiration in the head area, alternating chills and fever, and anxiety should be given *Chai-hu-kuei-chih-kan-chiang-tang* (Bupleurum, Cinnamon and Ginger Combination).

80. 傷寒五六日，頭汗出，微惡寒，手足冷，心下滿，口不欲食，大便鞕，脈細者，可與小柴胡湯。設不了了者，得屎而解。

Shang han [conditions] lasting five or six days with perspiration in the head area, mild chills, coldness of the hands and feet (two symptoms of lesser yin disease), congestion beneath the heart, loss of appetite (evidence of lesser yang disease), hard stools, and a small pulse may be treated with *Hsiao-chai-hu-tang* (Minor Bupleurum Combination). Recovery will occur when the bowel movements return to normal, [an effect of Minor Bupleurum Combination].

81. 傷寒五六日，嘔而發熱者，柴胡湯證具。而以他藥下之，柴胡證仍在者，復與柴胡湯，必蒸蒸而振，却發熱汗出而解。若心下滿而鞕痛者，大陷胸湯主之。但滿而不痛者，柴胡不中與之，宜半夏瀉心湯。

Here is a comparison of the herb prescriptions *Chai-hu-tang* (Bupleurum Combination), *Ta-hsien-hsiung-tang* (Rhubarb and *Kan-sui* Combination), and *Pan-hsia-hsieh-hsin-tang* (Pinellia Combination) in the treatment of *shang han* [conditions]. Shang han [conditions] of the *Chai-hu-tang* confirmation present vomiting and fever lasting five to six days even following purging by another herb. *Chai-hu-tang* initiates shivering followed by fever and perspiration which alleviates [the problem]. If there is congestion with hardness and pain beneath the heart, *Ta-hsien-hsiung-tang* (Rhubarb and *Kan-sui* Combination) is indicated. For cases with congestion beneath the heart without pain, *Pan-hsia-hsieh-hsin-tang* (Pinellia Combination) is recommended rather than *Chai-hu-tang* (Bupleurum Combination).

82. 太陽中風，下利嘔逆，其人漐漐汗，發作有時，頭痛，心下痞
鞭滿，引脇下痛，乾嘔短氣，汗出不惡寒者，十棗湯主之。

Chung feng [conditions] in greater yang disease are characterized by diarrhea and vomiting [due to water intoxication];
profuse perspiration [occurring] at regular intervals; headache; hardness, stagnancy, and congestion beneath the heart;
dragging [type of] pain below the ribs; retching; and rapid
respiration. (These symptoms represent a surface confirmation and should first be relieved before purgative herbs are
administered.) *Shih-tsao-tang* (Jujube Combination) is prescribed when perspiration occurs without severe chills.

83. 太陽病，醫發汗，遂發熱惡寒，因復下之，心下痞，按之濡，
其脈浮者，大黃黃連瀉心湯主之。心下痞，而復惡寒，汗出者
，附子瀉心湯主之。心下痞，與瀉心湯，痞不解，其人渴而口
燥，煩，小便不利者，五苓散主之。

Greater yang disease which has been treated by a physician
[first] with the sweating method and then with the purgation
method [due to mistaken diagnosis of inside confirmation]
will exhibit relapsing fever and severe chills [as a result of
administering incorrect herbs], hardness beneath the heart
with a sensation of tenderness [on palpation], and a floating pulse. This condition should be treated with *Ta-huang-
huang-lien-hsieh-hsin-tang* (Rhubarb, Coptis, and Scute Combination). Hardness beneath the heart, relapsing chills, and
perspiration should be treated with *Fu-tzu-hsieh-hsin-tang*
(Rhubarb and Aconite Combination). For patients in whom
the hardness is not relieved by *Hsieh-hsin-tang* (Pinellia Combination) and who experience thirst, dryness of the mouth,
anxiety, and dysuria, *Wu-ling-san* (Hoelen Five Herb Combination) is indicated.

84. 傷寒，汗出解之後，胃中不和，心下痞鞭，乾噫食臭，脇下有
水氣，腹中雷鳴下利者，生薑瀉心湯主之。

If, after the surface confirmation of *shang han* conditions has
been treated by the sweating method, there is continued
impairment of digestion, hardness beneath the heart, retching
that gives out a stench of food, fluid below the ribs, and
borborygmus with diarrhea, *Sheng-chiang-hsieh-hsin-tang*
(Pinellia and Ginger Combination) should be administered.

85. 傷寒中風，醫反下之，其人下利日數十行，穀不化，腹中雷鳴，
心下痞鞕而滿，乾嘔，心煩不得安，醫見心下痞，謂病不盡，
復下之，其痞益甚，甘草瀉心湯主之。

If [the surface confirmation] of *shang han* and *chung feng*
[conditions] are not relieved by treatment with the purgation method, there may be periods of diarrhea with undigested food each day, borborygmus, hardness, discomfort,
distress and congestion beneath the heart, retching, irritability, and uneasiness. If the physician, on observing such
congestion beneath the heart, erroneously regards it as being
due to an incomplete cure of the disease and institutes
another purgation method, the congestion will be aggravated.
Instead, for such a condition, *Kan-tsao-hsieh-hsin-tang*
(Licorice and Pinellia Combination) is indicated.

86. 傷寒，服湯藥，下利不止，心下痞鞕，服瀉心湯，已復以他藥，
下之，利不止，醫以理中與之，利益甚，赤石脂禹餘糧湯主之。

If incessant diarrhea, stagnancy, and hardness beneath the
heart have resulted following treatment with some purgatory
herb for the *shang han* condition further treated with Pinellia
formulas [such as *Kan-tsao-hsieh-hsin-tang* (Licorice and
Pinellia Combination), *Sheng-chiang-hsieh-hsin-tang* (Pinellia
and Ginger Combination) or *Pan-hsia-hsieh-hsin-tang* (Pinellia
Combination)] followed by even other purgatives and the
incessant diarrhea is further aggravated by the physician's
treatment with *Li-chung-tang* (Ginseng and Ginger Combination), the patient should then be mainly given *Chih-shih-
chih-yu-yu-liang-tang* (Kaolin and Limonite Combination).

87. 傷寒，發汗，若吐，若下，解後，心下痞鞕，噫氣不除者，旋
覆花代赭石湯主之。

If the sweating, vomiting or purgation method of treatment
has relieved the *shang han* [condition but] there is still hardness beneath the heart and hiccoughs, *Hsuan-fu-hua-tai-che-
shih-tang* (Inula and Haematite Combination) should be
given.

88. 太陽病，外證未除，而數下之，遂協熱而利，利下不止，心下
痞鞕，表裏不解者，桂枝人參湯主之。

When the surface confirmation of greater yang disease treated with the purgative method several times has not improved and there is a surface fever accompanied by diarrhea which is then followed by prolonged loose stools, hardness beneath the heart, and other unrelieved surface and inside symptoms, [the patient] should be treated primarily with *Kuei-chih-jen-sheng-tang* (Cinnamon and Ginseng Combination).

89. 病如桂枝證，頭不痛，項不強，寸脈微浮，胸中痞鞕，氣上衝咽喉，不得息者，當吐之，宜瓜蒂散 。

Diseases similar to those of the *Kuei-chih-tang* (Cinnamon Combination) confirmation without headache and stiffness of the neck but with a slightly floating pulse palpated on the *chun* location, hardness in the chest, congestion of the *ch'i* towards the pharynx, and labored respiration should be treated with the vomiting method and *Kua-ti-san* (Melon Pedicle Formula).

90. 傷寒，若吐若下後，七八日不解，表裏俱熱，時時惡風，大渴，舌上乾燥而煩，欲飲水數升者，白虎加人參湯主之 。

If *shang han* [conditions] treated by the [sweating], vomiting or purgation methods have not been relieved in seven to eight days and [symptoms appear of] internal fever spreading to the (body) surface, occasional mild chills, severe thirst with the desire to drink a tremendous amount of water, dryness of the tongue, and anxiety, [the patient should be treated mainly with *Pai-hu-chia-jen-sheng-tang* (Ginseng and Gypsum Combination)]. Ginseng is added to nourish and help replace the loss of body fluids due to use of sweating, vomiting, or purgation methods.)

91. 傷寒，無大熱，口燥渴，心煩，背微惡寒者，白虎加人參湯主之 。

Pai-hu-chia-jen-sheng-tang (Ginseng and Gypsum Combination) is advised for *shang han* [conditions] without "surface" fever but with dryness of the mouth, thirst (due to "inside" fever), disturbance of the heart, and mild chills of the back.

92. 傷寒，脈浮，發熱無汗，渴欲飲水，無表證者，白虎加人參湯主之 。

Pai-hu-chia-jen-sheng-tang (Ginseng and Gypsum Combination) should be prescribed for patients with *shang han* [conditions] with a floating pulse, fever without perspiration, and thirst, but with no "surface" confirmation. Those having a "surface" confirmation should never be treated with *Pai-hu-chia-jen-sheng-tang*.

93. 太陽與少陽合病，自下利者，與黃芩湯，若嘔者，黃芩加半夏生薑湯主之。

The combined confirmation of greater yang and lesser yang diseases that gives rise to diarrhea should be treated with *Huang-chin-tang* (Scute Combination). If vomiting is also present, *Huang-chin-chia-pan-hsia-sheng-chiang-tang* (Scute, Pinellia, and Ginger Combination) should be given.

94. 傷寒，胸中有熱，胃中有邪氣，腹中痛，欲嘔吐者，黃連湯主之。

Shang han [conditions] with fever in the chest [lesser yang disease], "evil force" (discomfort) in the stomach, abdominal aching, and a tendency towards vomiting should be treated primarily with *Huang-lien-tang* (Coptis Combination).

95. 傷寒八九日，風濕相摶，身體疼煩，不能自轉側，不嘔不渴，脈浮虛而濇者，桂枝附子湯主之。若其人大便鞕，小便自利者，去桂加白朮湯主之。

Patients with *shang han* [conditions] lasting eight to nine days due to a conflict between the [outside] wind and the [inside] moisture should be treated with *Kuei-chih-fu-tzu-tang* (Cinnamon and Aconite Combination). There will also be present generalized aching making movement difficult; a floating, weak, obstructed type of pulse (inside weakness); and an absence of vomiting and thirst. *Chu-kuei-chia-pai-chu-tang* (Aconite and Atractylodes Combination) is recommended for patients with hard (inspissated) stools and polyuria.

96. 風濕相摶，骨節疼煩，掣痛，不得屈伸，近之則痛劇，汗出短氣，小便不利，惡風不欲去衣，或身微腫者，甘草附子湯主之。

The conflict between the [outside] wind and the [inside] moisture due to the *shang han* condition as exhibited by aching of the joints; rapid respiration following perspiring; dysuria; mild chills; a disinclination to undress; occasional

27

mild generalized edema; and severe and painful muscular contractions in which the pain increases on light touch making movement difficult should be treated principally with *Kan-tsao-fu-tzu-tang* (Licorice and Aconite Combination).

97. 傷寒，脈浮滑，白虎湯主之。

Pai-hu-tang (Gypsum Combination) is indicated for *shang han* [conditions] of a floating and smooth pulse.

98. 傷寒解而後，脈結代，心動悸，炙甘草湯主之。

Shang han [conditions] that have been relieved [of fever] but have a continued knotted and irregular pulse and rapid heart palpitation should be given *Chih-kan-tsao-tang* (Baked Licorice Combination).

Summary

Article 1: Outlines the characteristic surface febrile confirmation of greater yang disease.

Article 2: Describes the *chung feng* condition as a mild form of the surface febrile confirmation of greater yang disease.

Article 3: Uses the term *shang han* to designate the severe form of the surface febrile confirmation of greater yang disease.

Article 4: Includes a discussion of *chung feng* conditions of greater yang disease with the *Kuei-chih-tang* (Cinnamon Combination) confirmation.

Article 5: Defines the *Kuei-chih-tang* (Cinnamon Combination) confirmation of greater yang disease.

Article 6: Outlines the *Kuei-chih-ko-ken-tang* (Cinnamon and Pueraria Combination) confirmation of greater yang disease.

Article 7: Describes how greater yang disease with a residual upward congestion treated with the purgation method may be treated with *Kuei-chih-tang* (Cinnamon Combination).

Article 8: Tells how the lack of response after three days of treatment with the sweating, vomiting, purgation, and acupuncture methods in greater yang disease is a result of improper therapy. The condition should be treated according to its pulse confirmation rather than as a normal confirmation.

Article 9: Characterizes the *Kuei-chih-chia-fu-tzu-tang* (Cinnamon and Aconite Combination) conformation of greater yang disease. This may represent an initial stage of lesser yin disease.

Article 10: Outlines the *Kuei-chih-chu-shao-yao-tang* (Cinnamon Minus Paeonia Combination) confirmation of greater yang disease. In contrast to the *Kuei-chih-chia-shao-yao-tang* (Cinnamon and Paeonia Combination) confirmation of greater yin disease which results because of mistreatment of greater yang disease, this confirmation may be considered as an unstable form of the *Kuei-chih-kan-tsao-tang* (Cinnamon and Licorice Combination) confirmation. Also included is a definition of the *Kuei-chih-chu-shao-chia-fu-tzu-tang* (Cinnamon, Ginger, and Aconite Combination) confirmation of greater yang disease.

Article 11: Delineates a case of greater yang disease with alternating chills and fever similar to that of lesser yang disease in order to explain the *Kuei-chih-ma-huang-ko-pan-tang* (Cinnamon and *Ma-huang* Combination) confirmation and to act as a warning for the *Hsiao-chai-hu-tang* (Minor Bupleurum Combination) confirmation.

Article 12: Discusses the reinforcement of the treatment of *Kuei-chih-tang* (Cinnamon Combination) confirmation with acupuncture.

Article 13: Tells how a second dose of *Kuei-chih-tang* (Cinnamon Combination) may be given to initially unresponsive cases with severe perspiration, a large pulse, and no thirst, in contrast to the *Pai-hu-chia-jen-sheng-tang* (Ginseng and Gypsum Combination) confirmation noted in Article 14. Also the use of *Kuei-chih-erh-ma-huang-i-tang* (*Ma-huang* and Double Cinnamon Combination) for malaria-like alternating chills and fever is differentiated from the use of *Kuei-chih-ma-huang-ko-pan-tang* (Cinnamon and *Ma-huang* Combination) as described in Article 11.

29

Article 14: Describes *Pai-hu-chia-jen-sheng-tang* (Ginseng and Gypsum Combination) confirmation, characterized by excessive perspiration, anxiety, and thirst following ingestion of *Kuei-chih-tang* (Cinnamon Combination). This reveals an initial stage of sunlight yang disease.

Article 15: States that greater yang disease in which the fever lasts longer than the chills is a surface weak confirmation with inside fever and may be treated with *Kuei-chih-erh-yueh-pei-i-tang* (Cinnamon, *Ma-huang,* and Gypsum Combination). This article is regarded as a warning about the use of *Ta-ching-lung-tang* (Major Blue Dragon Combination) discussed in Articles 23 and 24.

Article 16: Enumerates the residual symptoms following the use of *Kuei-chih-tang* (Cinnamon Combination) and the purgation method indicating the need for *Kuei-chih-chu-kuei-chia-fu-ling-pai-chu-tang* (Hoelen, Artactylodes, and Paeonia Combination). This condition also serves as a warning of the possibility of the *Chen-wu-tang* (Vitality Combination) confirmation of lesser yin disease.

Article 17: Describes how a quasi-*Kuei-chih-tang* (Cinnamon Combination) confirmation improperly treated with *Kuei-chih-tang* can convert successively into the following confirmations: *Kan-tsao-kan-chiang-tang* (Licorice and Ginger, Combination); *Shao-yao-kan-tsao-tang* (Paeonia and Licorice Combination); yang strong *Tiao-wei-cheng-chi-tang* (Rhubarb and Mirabillitum Combination), and absolute yin *Szu-ni-tang* (Aconite, Ginger, and Licorice Combination). This illustrates the importance of a definitive therapy for *shang han* (conditions) as even a minor, inappropriate treatment may result in progression through the various confirmations, the resultant condition becoming quite serious.

Articles 18 – 69: Following the discussion of *Kuei-chih-chia-ko-ken-tang* (Cinnamon and Pueraria Combination), these articles review first the normal and altered *Ko-ken-tang* confirmations, then the quasi-*Ma-huang-tang*

(*Ma-huang* Combination) confirmation, the inside fever of *Ta-ching-lung-tang* (Major Blue Dragon Combination) confirmation, *Hsiao-ching-lung-tang* (Minor Blue Dragon Combination) confirmation, and finally the altered confirmations - polydiaphoresis and oligodiaphoresis - after application of the sweating method. Discusses further the initiation of the disease process in the greater yang confirmation and the successive changes into lesser yang, sunlight yang, greater yin, lesser yin and absolute yin stages, ending with the *Szu-ni-tang* (Aconite, Ginger, and Licorice Combination) confirmation due to mistreatment. The importance of pulse diagnosis in the differentiation of these various confirmations from sunlight yang to absolute yin diseases is emphasized.

These articles (18-69) propound the main thesis on *shang han* conditions. They distinguish not only the greater yang pulse confirmation but show how it transforms into other diseases. For instance, greater yang disease treated by the sweating method with inadequate perspiration will gradually turn into lesser yang disease or alter to the greater yin confirmation. Further, the *Hsiao-chai-hu-tang* (Minor Bupleurum Combination) confirmation is differentiated from the *Kuei-chih-ma-huang-ko-pan-tang* (*Ma-huang* and Cinnamon Combination) confirmation. Two water congestion and three heat congestion formulas with *Chien-chung-tang* (Cinnamon and Paeonia Combination) and Gardenia formulas are also described. Alterations of lesser yang disease are discussed to illustrate how *Ta-chai-hu-tang* (Major Bupleurum Combination) is used for the transition from lesser yang to sunlight yang disease. The use of *Pai-hu-tang* (Gypsum Combination) is indicated when the disease transforms into the sunlight yang category and *Hsuan-wu-tang* (Vitality Combination) when it transfers to lesser yin disease. Finally, *Tao-ho-cheng-chi-tang* (Persica and Rhubarb Combination) and *Ti-tang-tang* (Rhubarb and Leech Combination) are specified in the presence of stagnant blood in greater yang

31

disease.

Articles
70—98:
These articles are concerned with disease conditions
in the chest and describe the major and minor *Chai-
hu-tang* (Bupleurum Combination) and similar confirmations. The first articles discuss stagnancy in the
chest and its developments which call for *Ta-hsien-
hsiung-tang* (Rhubarb and *Kan-sui* Combination) and
Hsiao-hsien-hsiung-tang (Minor Trichosanthes Combination). Article 77 reviews the *Chai-hu-tang* confirmation which is a complication of stagnancy of the
blood in a female who has suffered from a *chung feng*
condition for seven or eight days. The mild congestion and stagnancy in the chest lasting five or six days
are covered in Article 79. It emphasizes further that
Ta-hsien-hsiung-tang, Pan-hsia-hsieh-hsin-tang (Pinellia
Combination), and *Shih-tsao-tang* (Jujube Combination) confirmations should be differentiated from
Chai-hu confirmations, as well as *Chih-shih-chih-yu-
yu-liang-tang* (Kaolin and Limonite Combination),
Hsuan-fu-hua-tai-che-shih-tang (Inula and Haematite
Combination), and *Kuei-chih-jen-sheng-tang* (Ginseng
and Cinnamon Combination) confirmations from
various forms of *hsieh-hsin-tang* (purgatives). Articles
90 and 91 are quasi-*Pai-hu-chia-jen-sheng-tang* confirmations; article 92 is the *Pai-hu-chia-jen-sheng-tang*
confirmation. Finally, *Kua-ti-san* (Melon Pedicle
Formula), *Pai-hu-chia-jen-sheng-tang* (Ginseng and
Gypsum Combination), and quasi-purgatives such as
Huang-chin-tang (Scute Combination) and *Huang-
lien-tang* (Coptis Combination) confirmations are
described as warnings of sunlight yang disease. *Kuei-
chih-fu-tzu-tang* (Cinnamon and Aconite Combination), and *Kan-tsao-fu-tzu-tang* (Licorice and Aconite
Combination) confirmations of a semi-yin and semi-
yang class are similarly warnings of lesser yin disease.
This portion of the work concludes with directions
for the use of *Chih-kan-tsao-tang* (Baked Licorice
Combination) for *shang han* conditions where there is
continued palpitation and knotted and irregular pulse
after the fever has subsided.

Footnotes to Chapter One
1. See Glossary for explanation of the term "anemophobia".
2. See Appendix 6 on Malaria.

Chapter Two
Sunlight Yang Disease

99. 陽明之為病，胃家實是也。

The primary symptom of sunlight yang disease is fullness and discomfort in the abdomen.

100. 本太陽，初得病時，發其汗，汗先出不徹，因轉屬陽明也。

Greater yang disease treated with an [improper] sweating method may result in insufficient perspiration and change into sunlight yang disease.

101. 傷寒，發熱，無汗，嘔不能食，而反汗出濈濈然者，是轉屬陽明也。

Shang han [conditions] with fever but no perspiration, vomiting and loss of appetite [fall into the *Hsiao-chai-hu-tang* (Minor Bupleurum Combination) confirmation]. If excessive perspiration occurs, it is evidence that the disease has [partially] migrated to the sunlight yang stage.

102. 陽明病，若中寒者，不能食，小便不利，手足濈然汗出，必大便初鞕後溏。

Sunlight yang disease with inside chills (a symptom of absolute yin disease), loss of appetite, dysuria, and perspira-

tion of the hands and feet (quasi-sunlight yang symptoms)
will be accompanied by firm and then watery stools due to
weakness and coldness of the stomach which interferes with
water absorption. This is an absolute yin disease that is close
to sunlight yang disease.

103. 陽明病，脈遲，雖汗出，不惡寒者，其身必重，短氣，腹滿
而喘，有潮熱，手足濈然汗出者，大承氣湯主之。若汗多，
微發熱惡寒者，外未解也。其熱不潮，未可與承氣湯。若腹
大滿，不通者，可與小承氣湯，微和胃氣，勿令至大泄下。
Sunlight yang disease with a slow but strong pulse, perspiration but no severe chills, heaviness of the body [which
makes motion difficult], rapid respiration, stomach congestion, stridor [due to pressure in the chest], tide-[fluctuat-
ing] fever, and perspiration of the hands and feet should be
treated primarily with *Ta-cheng-chi-tang* (Major Rhubarb
Combination). Cases with excessive perspiration, mild fever
and severe chills indicate that the outside confirmation has
not been relieved. *Hsiao-cheng-chi-tang* (Minor Rhubarb
Combination) is given for stomach congestion with fullness
and for constipation in order to gently harmonize the
stomach function and guard against violent catharsis. *Ta-
cheng-chi-tang* (Major Rhubarb Combination) should not be
used as it may cause diarrhea.

   Warning: *Cheng-chi-tang* (Rhubarb Combination) should not
             be administered for febrile diseases other than
             the tidal type.

104. 陽明病，潮熱，大便微鞕者，可與小承氣湯。若不大便六七
日，恐有燥屎。欲知之法，少與小承氣湯，湯入腹中，轉失
氣者，此有燥屎也。乃可攻之。若不轉失氣者，此但初頭鞕
，後必溏，不可攻之。攻之必脹滿，不能食也。欲飲水者，
與水則噦。其後發熱者，必大便復鞕而少也。以小承氣湯和
之。不轉失氣者，慎不可攻也。
Hsiao-cheng-chi-tang (Minor Rhubarb Combination) may be
given for cases of sunlight yang disease with tide [fluctuat-
ing] fever and semi-solid stools. If no bowel movement
results after six or seven days, the stools have probably
become hard. Under these circumstances a small amount of
Hsiao-cheng-chi-tang may be administered. Once the disease
has affected the abdomen, gas may be passed, a sign of a

hard stool. Now the patient may be treated with the purgation method. Purgation is not recommended if no gas has been passed because the stools are hard but will become soft due to treatment with *Hsiao-cheng-chi-tang*. If the purgation method is utilized, stomach congestion and loss of appetite will result. Furthermore, if the patient is thirsty and drinks water, hiccoughs will occur. When fever is present, the patient often has firm and scanty stools and should be harmonized with *Hsiao-cheng-chi-tang* (Minor Rhubarb Combination). The purgation method is never advised in the absence of flatus.

105. 傷寒，若吐，若下後，不解，不大便五六日以上，至十餘日，日晡所發潮熱，不惡寒，獨語如見鬼狀，若劇者，發則不識人，循衣摸牀，怵惕而不安，微喘直視，讝語者，大承氣湯主之。

Shang han [conditions] that have not been relieved by the vomiting and purgation methods may exhibit an absence of bowel movements for five or six days, occasionally up to ten days, along with tide [fluctuating] fever at dusk without severe chills but with hallucinations. In severe cases the patient may fail to recognize others, be easily frightened, and have purposeless movements, restlessness, slight gasping respiration, fixed staring, and delirium. This indicates the need for *Ta-cheng-chi-tang* (Major Rhubarb Combination).

106. 陽明病，其人多汗，以津液外出，胃中燥，大便必鞕，鞕則讝語，小承氣湯主之。若一服讝語止者，更莫復服。

Sunlight yang disease, when present in a patient having a tendency to perspire severely even after a loss of body fluids, may manifest itself in dryness of the stomach (absence of gastric juices), hard stools, and delirium. This syndrome should be treated mainly with *Hsiao-cheng-chi-tang* (Minor Rhubarb Combination). The formula should be discontinued when the delirium subsides.

107 陽明病，讝語發潮熱，脈滑而疾者，小承氣湯主之。

Sunlight yang disease accompanied by delirium and tide fever suggests the *Ta-cheng-chi-tang* (Major Rhubarb Combination) confirmation, but if a smooth fast pulse is also present it is *Hsiao-cheng-chi-tang* (Minor Rhubarb Combination) confirmation.

108. 三陽合病，腹滿身重，難以轉側，口不仁，面垢，讝語，遺
尿，發汗則讝語甚，下之則額上生汗，手足逆冷，若自汗出
者，白虎湯主之。

A combination of the three yang diseases in which both the surface and inside have been affected resulting in poor circulation of the *ch'i* and blood may also exhibit abdominal distention; heaviness of the body; difficulty in movement; thirst and loss of taste; darkness of facial color; delirium; urinary incontinence; and, when treated with the sweating method, severe delirium. *Pai-hu-tang* (Gypsum Combination) should be administered to these yang disease patients who also show perspiration on the forehead, coldness of the hands and feet, or have spontaneous, generalized perspiration when treated with the purgation method.

109. 二陽併病，太陽證罷，但發潮熱，手足漐漐汗出，大便難而
讝語者，下之則愈，宜大承氣湯。

The complications of greater and sunlight yang diseases when the greater yang surface confirmation has been relieved but the sunlight inside confirmation continues to exhibit [the symptoms of] tide fever, severe perspiration on the hands and feet, constipation, and delirium will be relieved by the purgation method and *Ta-cheng-chi-tang* (Major Rhubarb Combiantion).

110. 陽明病，脈浮而緊，咽燥口苦，腹滿而喘，發熱汗出，不惡
寒，反惡熱，身重。若發汗則躁，心憒憒反讝語。若加溫針
，必怵惕煩躁不得眠。若下之則胃中空虛，客氣動膈，心中
懊憹，舌上胎者，梔子豉湯主之。若渴欲飲水，口乾舌燥者
，白虎加人參湯主之。若渴欲飲水，小便不利者，豬苓湯主之。

Sunlight yang disease when present in combination with the other two yang diseases will exhibit a floating, tense pulse (a confirmation of greater yang disease), dryness of the throat and a bitter taste in the mouth (a confirmation of lesser yang disease), abdominal distention with stridor, perspiration due to a fever, febriphobia instead of chillphobia, and a severe feeling of heaviness of the body (confirmation of sunlight yang disease). For cases of this type if the sweating method is applied, the patient will experience restlessness, mental confusion, and delirium [due to the loss of kidney fluids]. Restlessness and insomnia will occur if moxibustion is used. The purgation method removes the stagnancy in the stomach, but the harmful (diseased) ch'i then moves to the chest causing distress and also a coating on the tongue. These cases should be treated with Chih-tzu-shih-tang (Gardenia and Soja Combination). Cases in which thirst and dryness of the mouth and tongue are present should be given Pai-hu-chia-jen-sheng-tang (Ginseng and Gypsum Combination). Chu-ling-tang (Polyporus Combination) is recommended for patients with thirst and dysuria.

111. 陽明病下之，其外有熱，手足溫，心中懊憹，飢不能食，但頭汗出者，梔子豉湯主之。

Sunlight yang disease that has been treated by the purgation method but still exhibits external fever (remaining on the body surface), warm hands and feet, a sensation of distress in the chest, a feeling of hunger but no appetite, and perspiration on the forehead should be treated with Chih-tzu-shih-tang (Gardenia and Soja Combination).

112. 陽明病，發潮熱，大便溏，小便自可，胸脇滿不去者，與柴胡湯。

Sunlight yang disease with tide fever (a confirmation of sunlight yang disease), soft stools but normal urination, and protracted congestion in the chest (a residual confirmation of lesser yang disease) should be treated with Chai-hu-tang (Bupleurum Combination) in order to relieve the lesser yang confirmation. (This is done in accordance with this principle: Treat first the surface and then the inside.)

113. 陽明病，脇下鞕滿，不大便而嘔，舌上白胎者，可與小柴胡湯。上焦得通，津液得下，胃氣因和，身濈然汗出而解。

Sunlight yang disease [when present in combination with lesser yang disease] may exhibit hardness and congestion beneath the ribs, constipation (stagnancy in the lower warmer), vomiting (disharmony in the middle warmer), and white coating on the tongue (stagnancy in the upper warmer). Hsiao-chai-hu-tang (Minor Bupleurum Combination) is given to treat the upper warmer. When the upper warmer is normalized, the body fluids will then descend [and circulate in the triple warmer], and the stomach will be harmonized. The problem is usually resolved following marked perspiration.

114. 陽明中風，脈弦浮大，而短氣，腹都滿，脇下及心痛，久按之氣不通，鼻乾不得汗，嗜臥，一身及面目悉黃，小便難，有潮熱，時時噦，耳前後腫，刺之少差，外不解，病過十日，脈續浮者，與小柴胡湯，脈但浮，無餘證者，與麻黃湯。

The *chung feng* [condition] of sunlight yang disease [is a combination of the three yang diseases]. The symptoms are tension (lesser yang), floating (greater yang) and large (sunlight yang) pulse, rapid respiration, abdominal congestion (sunlight yang confirmation), pain beneath the ribs and aching over the precordium (lesser yang confirmation), difficulty in breathing when pressure is applied to the abdomen, dryness of the nose, lack of perspiration (greater yang confirmation), drowsiness, yellowish discoloration of the face and body (jaundice), difficulty in urination, tide fever, frequent hiccoughs, and swelling around the ears (lesser yang confirmation). If the swelling recedes following acupuncture but the outside symptoms linger for more than ten days with the floating pulse as before, then *Hsiao-chai-hu-tang* (Minor Bupleurum Combination) should be administered. *Ma-huang-tang* (*Ma-huang* Combination) is indicated for patients with no other symptoms but a floating pulse. (See Appendix 7 for further information on jaundice.)

115. 陽明病，自汗出，若發汗，小便自利者，雖鞕不可攻之。當須自欲大便，宜蜜煎導而通之。若土瓜根及大猪膽汁，皆可爲導。

Sunlight yang disease initially manifesting spontaneous perspiration that has been further treated with the sweating method and now exhibits polyuria should not be treated with purgatives in spite of the presence of hard stools. Constipation of this type is best treated with *Mi-chien-tao* (Mel Decoction Formula) alternated with the juice of snake gourd root (*Trichosanthes cucumeroides* Max.) or a big pig's gall.

39

116. 陽明病，發熱汗出者，不能發黃也，但頭汗出，身無汗，劑頸而還，小便不利，渴引水漿者，身必發黃，茵陳蒿湯主之。

Sunlight yang disease with fever and perspiration will not result in yellowish discoloration of the skin (jaundice). However, cases with perspiration on the head and neck areas only, difficulty in urination, and a tendency to drink a lot of fluids will ultimately end in jaundice. *Yin-chen-hao-tang* (Capillaris Combination) should be given.

117. 陽明證，其人喜忘者，必有畜血，屎雖鞭，大便反易，其色必黑，宜抵當湯，下之。

If the patient of the sunlight yang confirmation suffers from a loss of memory and has signs of stagnant blood and hard stools but no difficulty in moving the bowels, he should be treated by the purgation method along with *Ti-tang-tang* (Rhubarb and Leech Combination).

118. 陽明病，下之，心中懊憹而煩，胃中有燥屎者，宜大承氣湯。

If after treating sunlight yang disease with the purgation method there is [continued] general distress and distress in the heart and dry stools due to inside heat and firmness, *Ta-cheng-chi-tang* (Major Rhubarb Combination) should be given.

119. 大下後，六七日不大便，煩不解，腹滿痛者，此有燥屎也，宜大承氣湯。

For cases where after a marked purgation there is continued constipation of six to seven days due to loss of body fluids, unrelieved anxiety, abdominal fullness with pain (due to undigested and stagnated food) which is evidence of dry stools, *Ta-cheng-chi-tang* (Major Rhubarb Combination) is advised.

120. 食穀欲嘔者，屬陽明也，吳茱萸湯主之。

For cases of sunlight yang [confirmation] with a tendency toward vomiting after ingestion of food, *Wu-chu-yu-tang* (Evodia Combination) is indicated.

121. 太陽病三日，發汗不解，蒸蒸發熱者，屬胃也，調胃承氣湯主之。

Patients with greater yang disease lasting for three days who

have had incomplete relief following treatment with the
sweating method and who have a persisting fever due to
stomach trouble should be given *Tiao-wei-cheng-chi-tang*
(Rhubarb and Mirabilitum Combination).

122. 傷寒六七日，目中不了了，睛不和，無表裏證，大便難，身微
熱者，急下之，宜大承氣湯。

Shang han [conditions] that prevail for six to seven days
[the yang disease has progressed toward the yin stage] causing blurred vision, disturbed ocular function, absence of surface and inside confirmations [no lesser yang confirma-
tion], difficulty in defecation, and a mild body fever [firm
confirmation] should be purged without delay with *Ta-
cheng-chi-tang* (Major Rhubarb Combination).

123. 陽明少陽合病，必下利，脈滑而數者，有宿食也，當下之，
宜大承氣湯。

A combination of sunlight and lesser yang diseases with
diarrhea, smooth and rapid pulse, and undigested food
remaining in the stomach can be purged as an alternate
treatment with *Ta-cheng-chi-tang* (Major Rhubarb Combination).

124. 傷寒七八日，身黃如橘子色，小便不利，腹微滿者，茵陳蒿
湯主之。

Shang han [conditions] that have lasted for seven to eight
days with a yellow-orange coloration of the skin (jaundice),
dysuria, a tendency towards constipation, and mild congestion in the abdomen should be treated mainly with *Yin-
chen-hao-tang* (Capillaris Combination). For cases without
constipation *Yin-chen-wu-ling-san* (Capillaris and Hoelen
Five Formula) is recommended.

125. 傷寒，身黃，發熱者，栀子蘗皮湯主之。

Shang han [conditions] with a yellowish color of the skin
(jaundice) and fever should be given *Chih-tzu-po-pi-tang*
(Gardenia and Phellodendron Combination). This is a
type of jaundice of the *Yin-chen-hao* (Capillaris) confirmation.

41

126. 傷寒，瘀熱在裏，身必發黃，麻黃連翹赤小豆湯主之。

Shang han [conditions] with suppressed internal body fever [due to outside chills and inside moisture and heat] and a definite yellowish color of the skin should be treated primarily with *Ma-huang-lien-chiao-chih-hsiao-tou-tang (Ma-huang,* Forsythia, and Phaseolus Combination).

Summary

This chapter first outlines the symptoms of sunlight yang disease and then explains the use of *Ta-* or *Hsiao-cheng-chi-tang* (Major or Minor Rhubarb Combination) for firmness and congestion of the stomach and constipation. The 108th and following articles present illustrative cases that have not yet developed firmness of the gastrointestinal tract and explain why the purgation method should not be used. Next is described the different indications for *Chih-tzu-shih-tang* (Gardenia and Soja Combination); *Pai-hu-chia-jen-sheng-tang* (Ginseng and Gypsum Combination); *Chu-ling-tang* (Polyporus Combination); and *Hsiao-chai-hu-tang* (Minor Bupleurum Combination), the lesser yang confirmation of the constipated patient. It then discusses quasi-*Hsiao-chai-hu-tang* and quasi-*Ma-huang-tang* (*Ma-huang* Combination) confirmations, the related stomach congestion, constipation due to jaundice or stagnant blood, and the indications for *Yin-chen-hao-tang* (Capillaris Combination) and *Ti-tang-tang* (Rhubarb and Leech Combination). It further describes the *Wu-chu-yu-tang* (Evodia Combination) confirmation as a warning sign of lesser yin disease. The chapter concludes with a review of the use of *Chih-tzu-po-pi-tang* (Gardenia and Phellodendron Combination) and *Ma-huang-lien-chiao-chih-hsiao-tou-tang (Ma-huang,* Forsythia and Phaseolus Combination) for several types of yellowish discolorations of the skin (jaundice).

Chapter Three
Lesser Yang Disease

127. 少陽之爲病，口苦，咽乾，目眩也。

The primary symptoms of lesser yang disease [a condition characterized by being semi-surface and semi-inside], are a bitter taste in the mouth, dryness of the throat, and dizziness.

128. 少陽中風，兩耳無所聞，目赤，胸中滿而煩者，不可吐下，吐下則悸而驚。

Chung feng, a moderate and benign condition of lesser yang disease, is indicated by impaired hearing, redness of the eyes, and congestion and irritation in the chest. It should not be treated by the vomiting or purgation methods because they complicate palpitation and nervousness.

129. 傷寒脈弦細，頭痛發熱者屬少陽，少陽不可發汗。發汗則譫語。胃和則愈。

For *Shang han* conditions with a tense, small pulse, and headache and fever, which belong to the lesser yang confirmation, the sweating method is contraindicated. The condition may result in delirium if treated with the sweating

43

method. The patient may recover if the stomach is harmonized.

130. 本太陽病不解，轉入少陽者，脇下鞕滿，乾嘔不能食，往來寒熱。尚未吐下，脈沈緊者，與小柴胡湯。若已吐下，發汗，溫針，讝語，柴胡證罷，此爲壞病。

For patients with unrelieved manifestations of greater yang disease complicated by symptoms of lesser yang disease including hardness and congestion beneath the ribs, retching, loss of appetite, alternating chills and fever, and a sinking and tight pulse, *Hsiao-chai-hu-tang* (Minor Bupleurum Combination) is recommended if the vomiting or purgation methods have not been applied. If moxibustion, vomiting, or sweating methods have been used and there is delirium, it is of ominous import and indicates that the case has been mistreated. Now it is too late to institute the *chai-hu-chi* (bupleurum-containing formulas) as treatment.

Summary

This chapter includes only four articles which describe the formation, symptoms, and treatment of lesser yang disease. This by no means indicates that the lesser yang category is less significant, but the *chai-hu* (bupleurum), *hsieh-hsin-tang* (purgatives), and *chih-tzu* (gardenia) formulas useful in the treatment of lesser yang disease are discussed previously in the chapter on greater yang disease and so have not been repeated. Further, the section on greater yang disease was necessarily lengthy because of the inclusion of therapy applicable to all three yang categories as well as those of the yin diseases.

Chapter Four
Greater Yin Disease

131. 太陰之爲病，腹滿而吐，食不下，自利益甚，時腹自痛。若
下之，必胸下結鞕。

The primary symptoms of greater yin disease (the inside
disease of the three yin) are abdominal congestion, vomiting, loss of appetite, excessive diarrhea, and occasional
aching in the abdomen. Stagnancy and hardness in the chest
will occur if the case is treated by the purgation method
(due to a mistaken diagnosis of stagnancy in the abdomen).

Comparison of Greater Yin and Sunlight Yang Diseases

Greater Yin Diseases	Sunlight Yang Diseases
Inside chill confirmation	Inside fever confirmation
Weak abdominal congestion	Strong abdominal congestion
Weak pulse	Strong pulse
Diarrhea	Constipation
Treatment: nourishment	Treatment: purgation

132. 太陰病，脈浮者，可發汗，宜桂枝湯。

Both the sweating method and *Kuei-chih-tang* (Cinnamon
Combination), a formula for the surface fever confirmation

of greater yang disease, are recommended for patients with greater yin disease who have diarrhea, abdominal congestion, and a floating pulse (a symptom of surface fever).

133. 自利不渴者，屬太陰，其藏有寒故也，當溫之。
Diarrhea without thirst in greater yin disease is due to the chilling of the organs from poor metabolism and should be treated with warm formulas.

134. 本太陽病，醫反下之，因爾腹滿時痛者，桂枝加芍藥湯主之。大實痛者，桂枝加大黃湯主之。
Greater yang disease that should have been treated by the sweating method but instead was treated by the purgation method with resultant continued abdominal congestion and occasional aching should be given *Kuei-chih-chia-shao-yao-tang* (Cinnamon and Paeonia Combination). *Kuei-chih-chia-ta-huang-tang* (Cinnamon and Rhubarb Combination) is recommended for patients with constipation and abdominal stagnancy accompanied by severe pain [a symptom of sunlight yang disease]. The former is a greater yang formula and the latter is advised to absorb the yin.

Summary

This short chapter, as the one on lesser yang disease, consists of only four articles describing the manifestations of greater yin disease. Again here, as in the chapter on greater yang disease, overlapping formulas and additional data have not been repeated.

Chapter Five
Lesser Yin Disease

135. 少陰之為病，脈微細，但欲寐也。

The primary symptoms of lesser yin disease are a feeble and small pulse and a tendency towards drowsiness.

136. 少陰病，欲吐不吐，心煩但欲寐，五六日，自利而渴者，虛故引水自救。若小便色白者，少陰病形悉具。

The main characteristics of lesser yin disease include a tendency towards vomiting, anxiety, and drowsiness that lasts for five to six days followed by diarrhea; weakness; thirst and resultant intake of water to relieve this condition; and clear, undiluted urine.

137. 少陰病始得之，反發熱，脈沈者，麻黃細辛附子湯主之。

For patients contracting lesser yin disease with fever (a symptom of greater yang disease) and a sinking pulse, *Ma-huang-hsi-hsin-fu-tzu-tang* *(Ma-huang,* Aconite, and Asarum Combination) is indicated.

138. 少陰病，得之二三日，麻黃附子甘草湯，微發汗。

Lesser yin disease lasting for two to three days with no sign

47

of the inside confirmation should be treated with *Ma-huang-fu-tzu-kan-tsao-tang* (*Ma-huang*, Aconite, and Licorice Combination) to render mild sweating.

139. 少陰病，得之二三日以上，心中煩不得臥，黃連阿膠湯主之。

For lesser yin disease that persists for two to three days or more accompanied by anxiety and insomnia (an inside confirmation) *Huang-lien-ah-chiao-tang* (Coptis and Gelatin Combination) is the treatment.

140. 少陰病，得之一二日，口中和，其背惡寒者，附子湯主之。

Lesser yin disease that has lasted only one or two days with [a feeble and small pulse] and no dryness of the mouth but severe chills in the back should be treated primarily with *Fu-tzu-tang* (Aconite Combination).

141. 少陰病，身體痛，手足寒，骨節痛，脈沈者，附子湯主之。

Due to an inside chill confirmation, *Fu-tzu-tang* (Aconite Combination) is given to patients with lesser yin disease that exhibits generalized aching, chills of the hands and feet, aching of the joints, and a sinking pulse.

142. 少陰病，下利，便膿血者，桃花湯主之。

Lesser yin disease with diarrhea and suppurative, bloody stools should be treated with *Tao-hua-tang* (Kaolin and Oryza Combination).

143. 少陰病，二三日，至四五日，腹痛，小便不利，下利不止，便膿血者，桃花湯主之。

For lesser yin disease that has lasted from two to five days with aching of the abdomen due to inside chills, difficulty in urination, protracted diarrhea, and suppurative, bloody stools, *Tao-hua-tang* (Kaolin and Oryza Combination) is recommended. [This is a more severe problem than outlined in article 142].

144. 少陰病，吐利，手足逆冷，煩躁欲死者，吳茱萸湯主之。

Lesser yin disease characterized by vomiting, diarrhea, cold hands and feet, a feeble and weak pulse, and a severe anxiety of impending death should be given *Wu-chu-yu-tang* (Evodia Combination).

145. 少陰病，下利，咽痛，胸滿，心煩者，豬膚湯主之。

Chu-fu-tang (Pig's Hide Combination) is advised for cases of lesser yin disease with diarrhea (weakness of the lower warmer) without vomiting, coldness of the hands and feet, sore throat, congestion in the chest, and anxiety.

146. 少陰病，二三日，咽痛者，可與甘草湯。不差與桔梗湯。

Patients with lesser yin disease that has lasted two or three days who have a sore throat but no fever, diarrhea, and congestion in the chest should be given *Kan-tsao-tang* (Licorice Combination), or in case the desired result is not obtained *Chieh-keng-tang* (Platycodon Combination).

147. 少陰病，咽中傷生瘡，不能語言，聲不出者，半夏苦酒湯主之。

For patients suffering from lesser yin disease with throat problems due to inflammation and ulcers resulting in an inability to speak and a loss of voice, *Pan-hsia-ku-chiu-tang* (Pinellia and Vinegar Combination) is advised.

148. 少陰病，咽中痛，半夏散及湯主之。

Cases of lesser yin disease with a sore throat [which indicates an increase of yin and decrease of yang] should be treated with *Pan-hsia-san* (Pinellia Formula) or *Pan-hsia-tang* (Pinellia and Cinnamon Combination).

149. 少陰病，下利，白通湯主之。

Lesser yin disease with diarrhea should be treated mainly with *Pai-tung-tang* (Allium, Ginger, and Aconite Combination).

150. 少陰病，下利，脈微者，與白通湯。利不止，厥逆無脈，乾嘔煩者，白通加豬膽汁湯主之。

For patients with lesser yin disease with diarrhea and a feeble pulse, *Pai-tung-tang* (Allium, Ginger, and Aconite Combination) is advised. For protracted diarrhea, coldness of the limbs, and an almost imperceptible pulse, plus retching and anxiety, *Pai-tung-chia-chu-tan-chih-tang* (A.G.A.

49

and Pig's Bile Combination) is recommended.

151. 少陰病，二三日不已，至四五日，腹痛，小便不利，四肢沈重疼痛，自下利。其人或欬，或小便利，或不利，或嘔者，玄武湯主之。

Lesser yin disease persisting from two to five days with abdominal discomfort, difficulty in urination, heaviness and aching of the limbs, diarrhea, cough, excessive urination, constipation, and vomiting should be treated with *Chen-wu-tang* (Vitality Combination).

152. 少陰病，下利清穀，裏寒外熱，手足厥逆，脈微欲絕，身反不惡寒，其人面色赤，或腹痛，或乾嘔，或咽痛，或利止脈不出者，通脈四逆湯主之。

For patients with lesser yin disease who have diarrhea containing undigested food; inside chills and outside fever; coldness of the hands and feet; a feeble, weak, and dying-out pulse; severe chills; ruddy face; abdominal discomfort; retching; sore throat; and a nearly imperceptible pulse that does not change after a cessation of diarrhea, *Tung-mo-szu-ni-tang* (Aconite, Ginger, and Licorice Pulse Combination) is given.

153. 少陰病，其人或欬，或悸，或小便不利，或腹中痛，或泄利下重者，四逆散主之。

Lesser yin disease exhibiting coldness of the limbs, cough, palpitation, dysuria, abdominal aching, or tenesmus (unsuccessful straining to empty bowels or bladder) should be treated with *Szu-ni-san* (Bupleurum and *Chih-shih* Formula).

154. 少陰病，下利六七日，欬而嘔，渴，心煩不得眠者，猪苓湯主之。

Patients with lesser yin disease characterized by persistent diarrhea [causing loss of body fluids] for six to seven days, a cough, vomiting, thirst, anxiety, and insomnia should be treated with *Chu-ling-tang* (Polyporus Combination) [in order to moisten the dryness and dispel the fever].

155. 少陰病，得之二三日，口燥咽乾者，急下之，宜大承氣湯。

Cases of lesser yin disease that have lasted for only two to three days and that exhibit dryness of the mouth and throat indicating an abdominal and serious lesser yin condition should be purged immediately with *Ta-cheng-chi-tang* (Major Rhubarb Combination).

156. 少陰病，自利清水，色純青，心下必痛，口乾燥者，急下之，宜大承氣湯。

Immediate purging with *Ta-cheng-chi-tang* (Major Rhubarb Combination) is recommended for lesser yin disease with watery, clear, greenish color diarrhea; aching beneath the heart on palpation; and dryness of the mouth.

157. 少陰病，脈沈者，急溫之，宜四逆湯。

Lesser yin disease with a feeble, small, and sinking pulse (see Article 135) where the chill has entered the viscera should be warmed without delay and then treated with *Szu-ni-tang* (Aconite and G. L. Combination).

158. 少陰病，飲食入口則吐，心中溫溫欲吐，復不能吐，始得之，手足寒，脈弦遲者，不可下也。若膈上有寒飲，乾嘔者，不可吐也。當溫之，宜四逆湯。

The purgation method is not indicated for cases of lesser yin disease where there is vomiting following ingestion of water and food, discomfort in the chest, a tendency towards vomiting even without intake of fluids or food but an inability to do so due to the presence of chilly sputum, chills of the hands and feet, and a tense and slow pulse. The patient should be warmed with *Szu-ni-tang* (Aconite and G. L. Combination) rather than treated with the vomiting method, especially in cases with chilled sputum in the chest and retching.

Summary

First, Chapter Five enumerates the primary manifestations of lesser yin disease as chills, a feeble and small pulse, and a tendency towards drowsiness. Lesser yin disease with surface illness calls for *Ma-huang-hsi-hsin-fu-tzu-tang* (*Ma-huang* and

Asarum Combination) and *Ma-huang-fu-tzu-kan-tsao-tang* (Aconite, Licorice, and *Ma-huang* Combination). A review of fever originating from the chills of lesser yin disease which is treated with *Huang-lien-ah-chiao-tang* (Coptis and Gelatin Combination) is found next. The basic inside chill confirmation of lesser yin disease is then discussed, followed by illustrations of the uses of *Fu-tzu-tang* (Aconite Combination), *Tao-hua-tang* (Kaolin and Oryza Combination), *Wu-chu-yu-tang* (Evodia Combination), *Pai-tung-tang* (Allium, Ginger, and Aconite Combination), *Pai-tung-chia-chu-tan-chih-tang* (A.G.A. and Pig's Bile Combination), *Chen-wu-tang* (Vitality Combination), *Tung-mo-szu-ni-tang* (L. A. and Ginger Pulse Combination), and *Szu-ni-tang* (G. L. and Aconite Combination). Next, the confirmation of lesser yin disease with a sore throat is covered, together with a description of applicable prescriptions: *Chu-fu-tang* (Pig's Hide Combination), *Kan-tsao-tang* (Licorice Combination), *Chieh-keng-tang* (Platycodon Combination), *Pan-hsia-ku-chiu-tang* (Pinellia and Vinegar Combination), *Pan-hsia-san* (Pinellia Formula), and *Pan-hsia-tang* (Pinellia and Cinnamon Combination). Finally the use of *Szu-ni-san* (Bupleurum and *Chih-shih* Formula) for lesser yin conditions with *ch'i* stagnancy as well, as *Chu-ling-tang* (Polyporus Combination) and *Ta-cheng-chi-tang* (Major Rhubarb Combination) for fever following chills, is outlined. The chapter closes with a review of the alternating forms of lesser yin disease.

Chapter Six
Absolute Yin Disease

159. 厥陰之爲病，氣上撞心，心中疼熱，飢而不欲食，食則吐，下之，利不止。

The cardinal symptoms of absolute yin disease [a disease of yang within yin characterized by fever in the upper part of the body] are upward congestion towards the chest [greater yin disease is characterized by a downward congestion towards the abdomen], a sensation of hunger but no real desire for food, and vomiting of worms after ingestion of food.[1] If the purgation method is used for treatment, prolonged diarrhea will result.

160. 凡厥者，陰陽氣不相順接，便爲厥。

Absolute yin disease is an imbalance between yin and yang which causes coldness of the limbs.

161. 傷寒，脈微而厥，至七八日膚冷，其人躁，無暫安時者，非爲蚘厥也。令病者靜，而復時煩，須臾復止，得食而嘔，又煩，其人當自吐蚘，蚘厥者，烏梅圓主之。

Shang han conditions with a feeble pulse and coldness of

53

the limbs persisting for seven to eight days, followed by coldness of the skin, agitation, and restlessness, does not indicate the coldness of the limbs is due to intestinal worms but instead shows a marked case of organ coldness. The patient with worms appears quiet but has frequent attacks of discomfort that subside quickly (because the worm ascends up through the diaphragm]. If the patient experiences nausea following food intake, recurrent anxiety, and a vomiting of worms, the coldness of the limbs is due to worm infestation, an indication of absolute yin disease, and is best treated with *Wu-mei-yuan* (Mume Formula).

162. 傷寒脈滑而厥者，裏有熱，白虎湯主之。
Pai-hu-tang (Gypsum Combination) is recommended for *shang han* conditions manifesting a smooth pulse and coldness of the limbs due to "inside" fever.

163. 手足厥寒，脈細欲絕者，當歸四逆湯主之。若其人內有久寒者，宜當歸四逆加吳茱萸生薑湯。
Tang-kuei-szu-ni-tang (Tang-kuei and Jujube Combination) is recommended for patients with a sensation of chilled hands and feet [an outside weakness of yang] and with a small and weak pulse. This formula is given with *wu-chu-yu* (evodia) and *sheng-chiang* (fresh ginger) when the patient exhibits prolonged chills on the inside in addition to outside chills.

164. 大汗出，熱不去，內拘急，四肢疼，又下利厥冷而惡寒者，四逆湯主之。

Patients with severe perspiration resulting from inappropriate therapy, retention of heat within the body [a yin confirmation that has transformed from greater or sunlight yang disease], abdominal spasms, aching and coldness of the limbs, diarrhea, and severe chills should be treated with *Szu-ni-tang* (Aconite and G.L. Combination).

165. 大汗，若大下利，而厥冷者，四逆湯主之。
Patients with coldness of the limbs should be given *Szu-ni-tang* (Aconite and G.L. Combination) after being treated by the strong sweating method used for greater yang disease

or the vigorous purgation method used for sunlight yang disease.

166. 病人手足厥冷，脈乍緊者，邪結在胸中，心下滿而煩，飢不能食者，病在胸中，當須吐之，宜瓜蒂散。

Coldness of the hands and feet and a tight pulse indicate stagnancy in the chest. Congestion beneath the heart, anxiety, and a sensation of hunger with an inability to eat typifies an absolute yin condition in the chest. The patient should be treated by the vomiting method with *Kua-ti-san* (Melon Pedicle Formula).

167. 傷寒厥而心下悸，宜先治水。當服茯苓甘草湯。却治其厥。不爾，水漬入胃，必作利也。

Shang han conditions accompanied by coldness of the limbs and palpitation beneath the heart due to water toxin should be treated first for the water toxin. The patient should take *Fu-ling-kan-tsao-tang* (Hoelen and Licorice Combination) to increase the secretion and flow of urine, followed by a formula for coldness in the limbs. Otherwise, the stagnant water will go to the stomach, resulting in diarrhea.

168. 傷寒，本自寒下，醫復吐下之，寒格。若食入口即吐，乾薑黃芩黃連人參湯主之。

Shang han conditions that have been mistreated with an emetic or purgative because of misdiagnosis of inside chills for inside fever will result in chills that resist the fever at the upper warmer. *Kan-chiang-huang-chin-huang-lien-jen-sheng-tang* (Ginger and S.C.G Combination) to purge the fever and dispel the chills is prescribed if vomiting follows the ingestion of food.

169. 下利清穀，裏寒外熱，汗出而厥者，通脈四逆湯主之。

Tung-mo-szu-ni-tang (Aconite, Ginger, and Licorice Pulse Combination) is recommended for patients with diarrhea in which the stool has undigested food; abdominal chills; outside fever; perspiration; and coldness of the limbs.

170 熱利下重者，白頭翁湯主之。

Pai-tou-weng-tang (Anemone Combination) is advised for

patients with diarrhea due to inside fever and tenesmus.

171. 下利，腹脹滿，身體疼痛者，先溫其裏，乃攻其表。溫裏宜
四逆湯，攻表宜桂枝湯。

Cases with a combination of diarrhea, abdominal fullness
due to inside weakness and chills, and generalized aching [as
a result of surface fever] should be treated first for the
inside chills by warming with *Szu-ni-tang* (Aconite and G.L.
Combination) and then for surface (fever) by purging
with *Kuei-chih-tang* (Cinnamon Combination).

172. 乾嘔，吐涎沫，頭痛者，吳茱萸湯主之。

Wu-chu-yu-tang (Evodia Combination) is advised for patients with retching (weakness of the stomach), salivation (a
chill of the stomach), and headache (an insufficiency of
yang).

Summary

This chapter outlines the primary symptoms and confirmation of absolute yin disease. Illustrative cases of coldness of the
hands and feet as quasi-absolute yin disease are included. Other
examples of absolute yin disease are added for comparison: *Pai-hu-
tang* (Gypsum Combination) [confirmation] of limb coldness with
inside fever and the *Pai-tou-weng-tang* (Anemone Combination)
[confirmation] of diarrhea due to inside fever.

Footnote
1. See Appendix 8 for further explanation on worms.

Chapter Seven
Absolute Yin (*Huo Luan*) Disease[1]

173. 吐利，惡寒，脈微而復利，四逆加人參湯主之。
Vomiting, recurrent diarrhea, severe chills, and a feeble pulse should be treated with *Szu-ni-chia-jen-sheng-tang* (Ginseng, Aconite, and Licorice Combination).

174. 吐利，頭痛發熱，身疼痛，熱多欲飲水者，五苓散主之。寒多不用水者，理中丸主之。
Wu-ling-san (Hoelen Five Herb Formula) is indicated for patients with vomiting, diarrhea, headache, fever, generalized aching, and thirst. *Jen-sheng-tang* (Ginseng and Ginger Combination) is preferred for vomiting, diarrhea, inside chills, and a complete absence of thirst.

175. 吐利，汗出，發熱惡寒，四肢拘急，手足厥冷者，四逆湯主之。
Vomiting, diarrhea, perspiration, exhaustion of vitality, fever, severe chills, spasms of the limbs, and coldness of the hands and feet should be treated with *Szu-ni-tang* (Aconite and G.L. Combination).

176. 既吐且利，小便復利，而大汗出，下利清穀，內寒外熱，脈微
欲絶者，通脈四逆湯主之。

Tung-mo-szu-ni-tang (Aconite, Ginger, and Licorice Pulse Combination) is indicated for cases with vomiting, diarrhea containing undigested food (a result of exhaustion of body fluids), polyuria, excessive perspiration, inside chills, outside fever, and a feeble and dying-out pulse.

177. 吐巳下斷，汗出而厥，四肢拘急不解，脈微欲絶者，通脈四
逆加猪膽汁湯主之。

If vomiting and diarrhea have ceased but there is general exhaustion, cold perspiration (a severe chill condition of the body), spasms of the limbs, and a feeble and dying-out pulse, *Tung-mo-szu-ni-chia-chu-tan-chih-tang* (L. A., Ginger, and Pig's Bile Combination) should be given.

Summary

This chapter described patients with vomiting, diarrhea, and fever—a condition which resembles what is now known clinically as cholera. The symptoms of absolute yin disease and cholera are very similar, both exhibiting vomiting, diarrhea, and coldness of the hands and feet.

Footnote

1. See Appendix 9 for further information.

Chapter Eight
Post-Illness Relapses

178. 大病差後，勞復者，枳實梔子湯主之。

Chih-shih-chih-tzu-tang (*Chih-shih* and Gardenia Combination) is indicated following a serious illness where there is incomplete recovery of vitality and a chance for recurrence due to excessive physical and mental stress.

179. 傷寒，差以後，更發熱者，小柴胡湯主之。脈浮者，少以汗解之，脈沈實者，少以下解之。

Hsiao-chai-hu-tang (Minor Bupleurum Combination) is recommended for patients who have recovered from *shang han* [conditions] but are having relapses of fever. If the patient has a floating pulse (a confirmation of "surface" disease), a mild sweating agent with *Kuei-chih-tang* (Cinnamon Combination) is recommended. A mild purgation agent with *Tiao-wei-cheng-chi-tang* (Rhubarb and Mirabilitum Combination) is given to patients with a sinking solid pulse (inside firmness) for post-illness conditions.

180. 大病差後，從腰以下，有水氣者，牡蠣澤瀉散主之。
     Mu-li-tse-hsieh-san (Oyster Shell and Alisma Formula) is given to patients with edema below the waist following a serious illness.

181. 大病差後，喜唾久不了了，宜理中丸。
     Jen-sheng-wan (Ginseng and Ginger Formula) is recommended for patients with continued expectoration of thin sputum as a sequel to a serious illness.

182. 傷寒解後，虛羸少氣，氣逆欲吐，竹葉石膏湯主之。
     Chu-yeh-shih-kao-tang (Bamboo Leaf and Gypsum Combination) is advised following the relief of *shang han* [conditions] where there is continuing weakness, shallow respiration, upward congestion, and a tendency towards vomiting.

Summary

Several types of post-illness syndromes are discussed including those associated with *shang han* conditions.

Part II

A Study of the *Shang han lun*

by

Otsuka Keisetsu

Preface

I have devoted myself to the study of the *Shang han lun* for forty years during which period I have written a number of articles on the work. In addition, I explained this classic to students of Chinese medicine when I taught at the Takushioku University from 1937-1944. Also, since the Second World War (1941-1945) I have often discussed the book with young medical students studying medicine under my direction.

There is an old saying: "The study of Chinese medicine begins with the *Shang han lun* and ends with the *Shang han lun.*" I know I will wish to study this classic in detail all my life.

Recently there has been a growing tendency to study Chinese medicine, and those desiring to devote their time to the analysis of the *Shang han lun* are increasing in numbers. I do believe that the day will soon come when this ancient medical work will be accepted as part of modern medical theory. At the invitation of Mr. Hosaka Fujisore, chief editor of *Sogenshia*, I have been happy to translate the *Shang han lun* [into Japanese] with simple explanatory notes useful to the beginner. I hope it serves as an inspiration to clinical practitioners.

Most of the commentaries presently available on the *Shang han lun* are complicated and difficult to understand. I believe that my explanation of the work is rather simple. It is hoped that the neophyte will start from this compilation and then study the general commentary as he becomes more interested in the *Shang han lun.*

Chapter One
Introducing the *Shang han lun*

Among the Chinese medical classics, none can compare with the *Shang han lun* in the multiplicity of annotations and research studies written. This demonstrates not only the importance of the work but also the problems it presents. Our ancestral sages have already extensively discussed the volume from different aspects, a few examples of which follow.

The famous physician Wutsuki Kondai[1] of the Edo era of Japan was most generous in his praise of the *Shang han lun:* "No work more ingenious than this one has ever existed since the appearance of the universe. Who else but the sage (Chang Chung-ching) could have written it?"

Kitamura Kousou[2] said, "The *Shang han lun* is to medical science what the *Analects of Confucius* 論語 and the *Works of Mencius* 孟子 are to Confucianism." In other words, as Confucianism would have little meaning without these great works so Chinese medicine would have little meaning without the *Shang han lun*.

Nagatomi Dokshouan[3] went even further when he stated:
Those who wish to learn ancient medical science must first

63

extensively study the *Shang han lun* and then select a well-qualified physicain to work with as a friend and clinically test these principles. This may take five or even ten years but one must persist in his endeavors for success. This training will then serve as an adequate basis to review all subsequent revisions of the original work and to be able to decide which ideas are authentic or spurious and which are applicable to his endeavors, much like a mirror reflects the beauty or uncomeliness of a lady. Without such preparations, one could read hundreds of millions of medical books without understanding the art.

Dokshouan thus stressed the importance of reading the *Shang han lun* and the futility of random study. He also said, "It is unnecessary for the beginner in the field of medical science to examine much literature. It is enough to keep only one reference at the bedside—the *Shang han lun*." He also said, "The *Shang han lun* covers all diseases, and all diseases embrace the *shang han*." Dokshouan contends that the *Shang han lun* contained the principles governing the treatment of all illnesses and that the study of this great work acquaints one with the manifestations of disease. I agree with his statement that the *Shang han lun* explains the rules of variation of disease and the corresponding methods of treatment. No other medical treatise can compare with this king of all medical works, even though it presents many perplexities.

In spite of much research, the question of how the *Shang han lun* came to be remains unanswered and even the name of the author Chang Chung-ching remains an enigma. My research on this subject is the basis of this book. It was my personal opinion that the first step in the study of the *Shang han lun* would be to identify the various so-called originals from the spurious or adulterated texts that appeared in subsequent generations. I knew that this task would not be easy as many of my predecessors had done research in an attempt to verify the authenticity of the work and the author, but I followed a similar course and here present my opinions to the reader.

Footnotes

Chapter One

1. Wutsuki Kondai (1779-1848), also known as Yoshio or Kondai, was well versed in theology, Confucianism, Buddhism, Taoism, and medicine, hence his appellation of "Gosoksai". Some of his works are *Ku hsun i chuan* (Ancient Doctrines on Medicine) and *Ji pen i pu* 日本醫譜 (The Historical Register on Japanese Medicine).

2. Kitamura Kousou (1804-1876), also known as Chykuan Kousow as well as Kojou in his later years, wrote the *Shang han lu su yi* 傷寒論疏義 (An Explanation of the Essay on Different Diseases and Fevers) and *Chin kuei yao lueh su yi* 金匱要略疏義 (Explanation of the Summaries on Household Remedies).

3. Nakatomi Dokshouan (1732-1766), also known as Feng or Choyo or simply Dokshouan, was a disciple of Sankyo Toyo. Yoshimasu Todo thought him to be a despicable character, like an invisible enemy. He wrote *Man yu tsa chi* 漫遊雜記 (Random notes on Aimless Travels) and *Tu fang yao* (Research on Emetic Prescriptions).

Chapter Two
Chinese Medical Science
before the *Shang han lun*

Separation of Medicine from Witchcraft

China has the earliest developed culture in the world. However, due to the lack of historical records, the state of medical science prior to the Spring-Autumn Period (722-482 B.C.) is not known. According to legend, in the time of the Yellow Emperor (Huang Ti), prior to 722 B.C., there were many celebrated physicians including Chi Po 岐伯 , Lei Kung 雷公 , Kuei Yi-chu 鬼臾區 , Hsiao Shih 少師 , Hsiao Yu 少俞 , Ma Shi-huan 馬師皇 , Tung Chun 桐君 , Yu Fu 俞跗, Wu Peng 巫彭 , and Chi Po's teacher Chiu Tai-chi 僦貸季 , who mastered many individual branches of medicine. Wu Hsien 巫咸 became a well-known physician during the reign of Emperor Yao 堯 as did Prime Minister I Yin 伊尹 in the Yin dynasty. The latter describes methods of treating disease with decoctions in *Tang i lun* 湯液論 (A Discourse on Medical Decoctions and Liquids). Such narratives, which appeared in the Warring States Period, were no doubt inaccurate and difficult to believe. Historians, however, accepted these stories as true, such as that of Shen Nung 神農 , the god of husbandry, who supposedly tested the various herbs and founded medicine. The Yellow Emperor and Minister Chi Po

66

were reported to have established the principles of medicine. Recent research has proved that the legends of such people as San Huang Wu Ti 三皇五帝 (three emperors and five kings), Fu Hsi 伏羲 , Shen Nung 神農 , the Yellow Emperor, et al., as well as their contributions, were pure fabrications that appeared after the middle of the Warring States Period (403-221 B.C.).

The government subdivided medicine into four categories in the Chou dynasty; food, disease, ulcers, and veterinary — all headed by a different medical officer. This was duly recorded in the *Records of Etiquette* in the Chou dynasty 周朝 , leading some to believe that medicine had already been separated from witchcraft and prayers in the early Chou era. Shuno Choki[2], however, doubts that this is true, finding it difficult to believe that medical officers could divorce themselves from the sorcery so prevalent in this period. Hashimoto Soukichi[3] is also suspicious of the existence of the four officers.

It is written that the famous physician Pien Ch'iao of the Warring States Period once said, "Those who believe in sorcery instead of medicine cannot be cured." This indicates that although witchcraft and incantations were still widespread, the first signs of medical independence had appeared. Chinese medicine, prior to this period, therefore appears to be non-existent.

In the *Shan hai ching* 山海經 (Classic of the Mountains and Seas),[4] which is believed to be a work of the Warring States Period, it states that Wu Pen, Wu Yang, Wu Lu, and Wu Fen gathered the remains of those killed by a monster named Chi Yu and sprinkled them with some kind of medicinal in expectation of their revival, while others including Wu Hsien, Wu Chi, Wu Pan, Wu Pen, Wu Ku, Wu Chien, Wu Li, Wu Ti, Wu Hsieh, and Wu Luo explored the mountains in search of divine herbs. From this description, it is obvious that the witch also served as a physician and that medicine did not then exist as an independent profession.[5] The two became separated only after continued progress. Thus in ancient times, sorcery and medicine were indistinguishable. The division occurred in the Warring States Period of the Han dynasty and thereafter.

The Examination, Diagnosis, and Treatment Methods of Pien Ch'iao

Szu Ma-chien in the Han dynasty stated in his *Chin yueh-jen Pien Ch'iao chuan* 秦越人扁鵲傳 (Biography of Pien Ch'iao) under the section on "Biographies in the Historical Records" 史記列傳 : "Pien Ch'iao, whose surname was Chin and given name Yueh-jen, was from a place in what is now known as the province of Shantung." However, according to research carried out by Nakabi Bansan, the biography of Pien Ch'iao could not be regarded as entirely reliable as there were many noted physicians bearing the same name during the period from 700-300 B. C.

Szu Ma-chien's biography may have come about by collecting the various known legends without giving any criticism or comment. The information probably was modified and exaggerated, there being many controversial points. Nonetheless, it does contain a reasonably good outline of medicine as practiced during the Warring States Period. The diagnostic methods used by Pien Ch'iao were based primarily on observation and palpation of the pulses. Pien Ch'iao's saving of the like of the Prince of Kuo was a very famous legend and is cited in the very beginning of the "Preface" of the *Shang han lun.* The therapy employed was acupuncture and poison compresses (warm packs of liquid herbs).

There is also a story of Pien Ch'iao's meeting with the Marquis Huan of Chi. He said, "Your majesty's illness appears to be in the muscles. If it is not treated, it might get worse." The Marquis replied, "I have no sickness." When Pien Ch'iao left, Huan told his subjects, "Physicians are always self-seeking. They treat healthy people in order to demonstrate their merit." Five days later Pien Ch'iao again met with the Marquis and said, "Your majesty is sick and the condition lies in the blood vessels. It might become worse without treatment." The Marquis said, "I am quite all right." The Marquis was again displeased after Pien Ch'iao's departure. A further interview with the Marquis took place five days later. Pien Ch'iao repeated, "Your highness is ill. The illness lies between the stomach and the intestines. It might become worse without treatment." The Marquis did not respond but obviously was so upset that Pien Ch'iao left. Pien Ch'iao on meeting with the Marquis after another five day interval took one look and left. The Marquis then sent someone to ask why he had suddenly departed. Pien Ch'iao responded, "When the sickness lies in the muscles, it can be cured by moist compresses; when it is located in the vessels, it can be treated with acupuncture; when it rests in the stomach and intestines, it can be improved with wine and unstrained liquor; but when it invades the bone marrow, it cannot be ameliorated even by God who controls all life and death. Now that your majesty's illness has reached the bone marrow, there is nothing I can do to help. That is why I did not request permission to treat your majesty." Five days later the Marquid became ill and sent for Pien Ch'iao. Unfortunately he had already left, and the Marquis soon died.

From the above description, one has a rough impression of the methods of medical treatment utilized by Pien Ch'iao. However, by way of comparison, it is quite different from that used in the *Shang han lun.* This was due to the fact that Chinese medicine was not yet separated from witchcraft in Pien Ch'iao's time. Advancements in medicine were not apparent until the end of the Warring States Period (320-250 B.C.), and these were furthered in the Chin and Han dynasties[6]. The *Huang ti nei ching* 黃帝內經 and the *Shang han lun* are the two classics that represent the apogee of medicine in the Han dynasty.

Ch'un-yu I and Hua To 淳于意與華佗

There is a biography in the Historical Records 史記列傳 on the celebrated physician Ch'un-yu I, who practiced medicine during the reign of Emperor Wen in the early Han period. His diagnostic and therapeutic methods are discussed. The following story is recorded. Ch'un-yu I, or Ts'ang Kung as he was more familiarly known, came from the same country, Chi, as Pien Ch'iao (Ch'in Yueh-jen). He studied the *Huang ti nei ching* 黃帝內經 and Wang Shu-ho's *Moching* 脈經 (Pulse Classic) under the well-known physician Kung-ch'eng Yang-ching. He relied primarily on the pulses for diagnosis, and acupuncture and moxibustion for treatment. The use of herbs in the form of decoctions was less frequently employed. At present the only information that we have available on the medical technique utilized by Ch'un-yu I is derived from the Historical Records. There is no further knowledge of his medical pursuits except for writings of Pan Ku 班固 in the Later Han dynasty where he briefly mentions in his *Han shu i wen chih* 漢書藝文志 (Record of Books, Techniques, and Literature of the Han Dynasty), "In most ancient times we had Chi Po and Yu Fu; in the middle period, Pien Ch'iao and Chin Ho. Then down to the Han dynasty we had (only) Ts'and K'ung (Ch'un-yu I) whose techniques are now unknown."

At the end of the Later Han dynasty, there was another physician named Hua To whose work became known through the *Ho han shu* 後漢書 (Books of the Later Han Dynasty), *Fang shu lieh chuan* 方術列傳 (Biographies on Medical Techniques), *San kuo chih* 三國志 (The Story of the Three Kingdoms), *Hsiang yang fu chih* 襄陽府志 (The History of Hsiang Yang fu), and *Hua to chuan* 華佗傳 (The Biography of Hua To). These references show that Hua To, also known as Yuen Hua, specialized in surgery and was widely known for his abdominal operations carried out with *Ma-fei-san* 麻沸散 , an anesthetic. He was well versed in mental health and he maintained his youthful appearance until he reached the age of 100. Among his disciples, there were two important ones, Wu Pu 吳普 and Fan Ar 樊阿 . The former was taught the five styles of Chinese exercises, the so-called "Five Beasts' Play."[7] These were also known as Guidance Techniques. Fan Ar was trained in the use of the prescription *Chi-yeh-ching-nien-san*[8] 漆葉青黏散 which in prolonged administration was purported to lengthen life up to one hundred years without any greying of the hair. Hua To was said to have studied methods of divinity. Legend says that he used only a very few herbs and a small number of points for acupuncture and moxibustion.

It is thus apparent that the methods of diagnosis and treatment employed by Ch'un-yu I and Hua To varied considerably from those recorded in the *Shang han lun,* indicating completely different origins.

Medical Books Used Before the *Shang han lun*

Since the evidence demonstrates that the physicians previously discussed practiced medicine that differed from that recorded in the *Shang han lun,* it would be natural to ask what medical works were available prior to this classic.

The following bibliography is found in the section "The Record of Techniques and Literature" 藝文志 in the *Books of the Han Dynasty* 漢書 compiled by Pan Ku in the Later Han period. It includes the various medical treatises that were in existence up to ca. A.D. 100. These are divided into the following categories: "Medical Classics"[9] 醫經 - seven schools of thought contributing 216 volumes; "Classics and Formulas"[10] 經方 - eleven systems comprising 274 works; "Bedroom Arts"[11] 房中 - eight documents composed of 186 essays; and "Divinity"[12] 神還 - ten creeds incorporating 205 tracts. A detailed list of these volumes follows.

Medical Classics

Title	Amount	Condition
Huang ti nei ching 黃帝內經 (Yellow Emperor's Classic of Internal Medicine)	18 volumes	destroyed
Wai ching 外經 (Yellow Emperor's Classic of External Medicine)	37 books	lost
Pien Ch'iao's Nei ching 扁鵲內經 (Pien Ch'iao's Classic of Internal Medicine)	9 tomes	lost
Wai ching 外經 (Pien Ch'iao's Classic of External Medicine)	12 monographs	lost
Pai's Nei ching 白氏內經 (Pai's Classic of Internal Medicine)	38 manuals	unavailable

71

Title	Amount	Condition
Wai ching 外經 (Pai's Classic of External Medicine)	36 tracts	lost
Pang ching 旁經 (Branch Classic)	25 volumes	lost

Classics and Formulas

五藏六府痺十二病方
Wu tsang liu fu pi shih erh ping fang
(Formulas for the Twelve Diseases of Palsy with the Five Solid and Six Lumenal Viscera) — 30 volumes — lost

五藏六府疝十六病方
Wu tsang liu fu shan shih liu ping fang
(Formulas for the Sixteen Diseases of Hernia of the Five Solid and Six Lumenal Viscera) — 40 volumes — missing

五藏六府痺十二病方
Wu tsang liu fu pi shih erh ping fang
(Formulas for the Twelve Diseases of Palsy of the Five Solid and Six Lumenal Diseases) — 40 tomes — lost

風寒熱十六病方
Feng han jeh shih liu ping fang
(Formulas for the Sixteen Diseases due to Wind, Cold, and Fever) — 26 monographs — missing

72

Title	Amount	Condition
Chin shih huang ti pien chiao yu fu fang 秦始皇帝扁鵲俞跗方 (Emperor Shih of Chin's *Pien Ch'iao* and Yu Fu Formulas)	23 treatises	non-extant
五藏傷中十一病方 *Wu tsang shang chung shih i ping fang* (Formulas for the Eleven Diseases due to Internal Injuries to the Five Solid Viscera)	31 tracts	lost
客疾五藏狂顛病方 *Ke chi wu tsang kuang tien ping fang* (Formulas for Epilepsy and Mania due to Involvement of the Five Solid Viscera)	17 volumes	unavailable
金創瘲瘛方 *Chin chuan chung chi fang* (Formulas for Knife Wounds and Infantile Convulsions)	30 books	missing
婦人嬰兒方 *Fu jen ying erh fang* (Formulas for Women and Children)	19 volumes	lost
湯液經方 *Tang i ching fang* (Classical Formulas of Decoctions and Liquids)	32 tomes	missing
神農食禁 *Shen nung shih chin* (Shen Nung's Food Incompatibilities)	7 monographs	missing

Title	Amount	Condition

Bedroom Arts

Zon Chen's yin tao 容成陰道
(Zon Chen's Female Ways) — 26 tomes — missing

Wu Chen-tzu yin tao 務成子陰道
(Wu Chen-tzu's Female Ways) — 36 treatises — missing

Yao shun yin tao 堯舜陰道
(Emperor Yao and Shun's Ways
of Women) — 23 tracts — unavailable

湯盤庚陰道
Tang pan ken yin tao
(Pan Ken's Female Ways – Tang
Dynasty) — 25 monographs — lost

天老雜子陰道
Tien lao tsa tzu yin tao
(Tien Lao Tsa Tzu's Ways of
Women) — 20 volumes — missing

Tien i yin tao 天一陰道
(Tien I's Female Ways) — 24 works — lost

黃帝三王養陽方
*Huang ti san wang yang yang
fang*
(The Yellow Emperor's and
Three Kings' Aphrodisiac Form-
ulas) — 20 books — lost

三家內房有子方
San chia nei fang yo tzu fang
(Three Schools' Bedroom For-
mulas for Fertility) — 17 tomes — non-extant

Title	Amount	Condition

Divinity 神僊

宓戲雜子道
Mi shih tsa tzu tao
(Mi Shih's Miscellaneous Ways)

20 chapters — unavailable

上聖雜子道
Shan Sheng tsao tzu tao
(Shan Sheng's Miscellaneous Ways

26 treatises — missing

道要雜子道
Tao Yao Tsa Tzu tao
(Essentials of Taoism: the Miscellaneous Ways)

28 tracts — missing

黃帝雜子步引
Huang ti tsa tzu pu yin
(The Yellow Emperor's Introduction to the Miscellaneous Ways)

12 volumes — lost

黃帝岐伯按摩
Huang ti chih po an mo
(The Yellow Emperor's and Chih Po's Massages)

10 monographs — non-extant

黃帝雜子芝菌
Huang ti tsa tzu chih chun
(The Yellow Emperor's Miscellaneous Knowledge and Guide to Uses of Mushrooms)

18 works — non-extant

黃帝雜子十九家方
Huang ti tsa tzu shih chiu chia fang
(The Yellow Emperor's Miscellaneous Knowledge Concerning 19 Schools' Formulas)

19 schools contributing 21 books — unavailable

75

Title	Amount	Condition
泰一雜子十五家方 *Tai i tsa tzu shih wu chia fang* (Tai I's Miscellaneous knowledge Concerning 15 Schools' Formulas)	15 schools contributing 22 treatises	missing
神農雜子技道 *Shen Nung tsa tzu chi tao* (Shen Nung's Miscellaneous Feasts and Ways)	23 volumes	non-extant
泰一雜子黃治 *Tai i tsa tzu huang chih* (Tai I's Miscellaneous Methods of the Ways of the Yellow Emperor)	31 tracts	lost

All of the foregoing books have been lost completely with the exception of the *Huang ti nei ching*. These classics, however represent the resources upon which the *Shang han lun* was based.

Wutsuki Kondai in his *Ku shun i chuan* 古訓醫傳 (Ancient Doctrines on Medical Science) contends that the *Shang han lun* as we know it today was comparable to the *Feng han jeh shih liu ping fang* 風寒熱十六病方 (Formulas for the Sixteen Diseases due to the Wind, Cold and Fever) as recorded in Pan Ku's *Record of Books, Techniques, and Literature*. It is unfortunate but there is no research information available to support this supposition.

Footnotes to Chapter Two

1. Soukichi, Hashimoto; *Tung yang wen hua shih ta shih* 東洋文化史大系 (The Great System of Oriental Culture).

Volume 1. Chapter on "The Mythological and Legendary Age."

2. Choki, Shuno; *Chi na hsueh wen shu* 支那學文藪 (An Assembly of Chinese Literature). Addendum to "Continuation on Witchery".

3. Soukichi, Hashimoto; *Tung yang wen hua shih ta shih* 東洋文化史大系 (The Great System of Oriental Culture) Volume 1. Chapter on "Legends About the Initial Chou".

4. Kokawa, Takuchi in his *Chi na li shih ti li yen chiu* 支那 歷史地理研究 (A Study on Chinese History and Geography) contended that the *Shan hai ching* was written during the Warring States Period and that there were many errors in the text.

5. Choki, Shuno; *Chi na hsueh wen shu* 支那學文藪 (An Assembly of Chinese Literature). Addendum to "Continuation on Witchery."

6. Shih Hu; *Chung kuo che hsueh lun* 中國哲學論 (A Treatise on Chinese Philosophy).

7. The Five-Beasts' Play was one type of guidance technique in which the exerciser mimicked the movements of the tiger, deer, bear, monkey, and bird as a form of exercise and self-massage. Further data on this method can be found in *Huang han i hsueh chi tao yin chi shih teh kao cha* 皇漢醫學及導引之史 的考察 (Chinese Medicine and Investigation into the History of Guidance Techniques by Ishihara Boshu.)

8. This prescription is also known as *Nien-ti-chieh* (*Polygonatum officinale* A.) or *Huang-chih* (*Polygonatum falcatum* A. Gr). It is listed in the *Shen nung pen ts'ao ching* 神農本草經 (Shen Nung's Herbal Classic) as being sweet or bland tasting and indicated primarily for the five toxins of the heart and abdomen; it is of benefit to the *ch'i* of the spleen, spiritually and mentally tranquilizing, heart calming, and harmonizing. Extended use of this herb makes the body light and youthful and lengthens one's life akin to the gods.

9. One reads in the *Record of Books, Techniques, and Literature* of the Han dynasty that the medical classics were concerned with the blood, the blood vessels, longitudinal and latitudinal meridians, bones, marrow, yin (female principle), yang (male principle), "surface" and "inside" with respect to the cause of the disease, the differentiation of life from death, the treatment of disease by means of stone needles (acupuncture), decoctions, and fire (moxibustion). Herbal formulas were prescribed according to

their properties in order to initiate the proper action, much like a magnet attracts iron. The natural properties of herbs were recognized. However, it was felt that the poorly trained practitioner could mistake alleviation in the patient for aggravation, and surviving for dying.

10. Classical formulas were given according to the cold or warm properties of the herbs, the action of stone needles (acupuncture), the severity of the illness, the nourishing action of herbs, the interaction of ch'i (vitality) and herbs, and the differences among the five bitter and six acrid flavors. They were intended to produce favorable reactions between fire and water in order to relieve obstruction, improve constipation, and allow recovery of the patient. Those who improperly treated the patient used hot herbs for hot diseases or cold herbs for cold diseases. As a consequence, vitality and vigor were injured internally, a condition not evident from the outside. If this occurred it was solely the fault of the physician.

11. The Bedroom Arts represent a science that is concerned with temperament and ways to control the desires and supress inner sensuality by following the way of the sages: restraint. In the records of literature it says music was also employed by the ancestral kings to soothe the pressures of daily affairs. If pleasures are curbed with appropriate temperance, one will be calm and live long. Also if one is overindulgent without considering the result, one will become prone to disease and die as a consequence.

12. Divinity is concerned with the ways of preserving spiritual life while pursuing the leisure arts of the outside world. The purpose is to have a calm, peaceful mind without worry or fear and to regard life and death as being equally significant. However, if one devotes his or her entire life to this premise, one can easily fall into error and misconstrue the wisdom of the holy sages by becoming a hermit. As Confucius said, "There are records describing the hermetic life and singular existence in previous generations, but I do not do so myself."

Chapter Three
The Appearance of the *Shang han lun*

Shang han lun and Chang Chung-ching

The authorship and date of the *Shang han lun* has long intrigued researchers. It has been conceded, generally, that it was composed by Chang Chung-ching in the late Eastern Han dynasty. The book contains a review of all prior works on effective prescriptions and medical techniques. Several questions concern us: first, who is the writer Chang Chung-ching; and second, how did the work come to be written.

First, we will discuss Chang Chung-ching. He has been thought to have lived during the late Eastern Han dynasty. A biography of Hua To (A.D. 110-207), a famous physician, who was active from the end of the latter Han era to the Three Kingdom's Period is included in the histories of these eras but there is no mention of Chang Chung-ching. From this Gihaku Furuya[1] concluded that Chang Chung-ching was a fictitious name, but he could present no conclusive supportive evidence that he did not exist.

Lin Yi wrote the introduction to the *Shang han lun* that was printed in the Sung dynasty. He quoted a text from *Ming yi lu* (The Record of Famous Physicians) and gave this information on Chang Chung-ching's life: "There is no biography of Chang Chung-

79

ching in the *Hou han shu* (History of the Eastern Han Dynasty), but he was thought to have been an inhabitant of Nan Yang. His name was Chi; Chung-ching was an alias. He was enrolled initially as a *Shao lien* and subsequently became the magistrate of the Changsha Prefecture. At a young age he became a pupil of Chang Po-tzu in his native town. However, his contemporaries soon felt his art in using prescriptions and medical techniques surpassed those of his teacher". Unfortunately, the *Ming yi lu* has been lost so we have no information concerning its author or date of publication.

The name Chang Chi is not included in the official list of those who served as magistrate of the Changsha Prefecture at the end of the Han dynasty, only a person named Chang Hsien who was killed by Sun Chien of Wu in the Three Kingdoms Period.[2] These two individuals are not, obviously, the same person. It is doubtful, also, if Chang Chi and Chang Chung-ching are the one and the same.

Chiukei Chiotani thought that Chang Chung-ching and Hua To were contemporaries but that Chang Chi lived a little later. However, he presented no evidence to support his conclusions or to refute the data in the *Ming yi lu*[3].

Some additional material on Chang Chung-ching of the Eastern Han dynasty and Three Kingdoms Period is found in the preface of the *Chia yi ching* (Classic of Medical Fundamentals) by Huang-fu Mi. This is fully quoted in *Chun i wen kuan chang chung ching i hsueh* (A Review of Chang Chung-ching's Medical Science from the Lost Books) with an explanation.[4] The story told is that Chang Chung-ching recommended *Wu-shih-san,* a Chinese herbal prescription, to Wang Chung-hsuan when Wang was in his early twenties. Wang died at forty-one, two decades later in the twenty-second year of the Chien An Period during the reign of Emperor Hsien in the Han dynasty. This means that Chang Chung-ching prescribed *Wu-shih-san* to Wang in the second year of the Chien An era. In the preface of the *Shang han lun,* the author says that he wrote it before the tenth year of Chien An. We can infer, therefore, that it was the eighth or ninth year of this time. (This appears to be an error as will be noted later.) It does imply, however, that *Wu-shih-san* was his favorite prescription before he composed the *Shang han lun* and that his methodology was prophetical. This is a key point important to the understanding of Chang Chung-ching's medical practice. (The medical viewpoint in the original copy of the *Shang han lun* differed from what Chang Chung-ching practiced. This represents proof material which will be discussed subsequently.) The *Tai ping yu lan* (Encyclopedia Read by Emperor of the Tai Ping Era) also tells of giving *Wu-shih-san* to Wang. However, this work and the *Chia yi ching* differ in relation to his age. Huang-fu Mi was three when Wang died in the second year of the Chien An era; therefore, his information was no doubt derived from oral transmission of Chang's contemporaries, lending greater credence to the data given in the *Chia yi ching*. There are, however, those who are still skeptical as to whether or not the preface of the *Chia yi ching* was written by Huang-fu Mi.

Wang Ping, who lived in the period of Pao Ying (A.D. 262) T'ang dynasty, in the preface of his commentary on the *Su wen*[5] (Simple Questions) mentioned that there was a famous physician of the era from the late Eastern Han to the Wei dynasty (one of the Three Kingdoms) called Chang Chung-ching. He said, "Master Chung Yu in the Han dynasty and Masters Chang (Chang Chung-ching) and Hua in the Wei reign were known to have understood the real essence of medical science."

Dating of the *Shang han lun*

Professor Tamehito Okanishi in his *Sun i chien i chieh kao* (A Research on the Medical Books Prior to Sung Dynasty) stated that Chang Chung-ching's *Ping ping yao fang* (A Comment on Diseases and Important Formulas) in one volume and his *Pien shang han* (The Identification of Fever Diseases) in ten volumes were already in print in the Liang Dynasty (A.D. 464-549). We further find in the *Ching chieh chih* (Gazette of Classics) under the "History of Sui Dynasty" (A.D. 589-618). "In Liang there was *Ping ping yao fang* (A Comment on Diseases and Important Formulas) by Chang Chung-ching, one volume, and there was *Pien shang han* by Chang Chung-ching, 10 volumes, lost." The contents of *Ping ping yao fang* is not now known but *Pien shang han* appears to be identical to that of the *Shang han lun* as we know it today. This seems to indicate that there was a book called *Pien shang han* in ten volumes by Chang Chung-ching in the period A.D. 500-550, but it seems to have been lost in the Sui dynasty

(A.D. 589-618). Also in the *Ching chieh chih* (Gazette of Classics) under the "History of the Sui Dynasty" there was a bibliography of books in which was found *Chang Chung-ching's Prescriptions*, fifteen volumes. In addition, Wang Shu-ho's *Chang Chung-ching's Prescriptions*, fifteen volumes, is listed in the *Ching chieh chih* (Gazette of Classics) of the old *Histories of the T'ang Dynasty* (A.D. 618-907). This proves that Wang Shu-ho's *Chang Chung-ching's Prescriptions* in fifteen volumes and *Pien shang han* in ten volumes existed in the T'ang dynasty.

Here one point calling for special attention is that the character *tsu* (卒) in the name *Shang han tsu ping lun* was regarded by Taki Rekiso and other famous scholars as a misrepresentation of the character *tsa* (雜). In fact *tsu* (卒) is the correct character. This will be discussed later.

The above discussion gives an idea of some of the problems concerning the origin and development of the *Shang han lun* and the life of Chang Chung-ching. It seems fairly well established then that the *Shang han lun* existed ca. A.D. 500.

The Completion of the *Shang han lun*

Why was the *Shang han lun* written? What is its structure? Let us refer to the preface of this monumental work. "My relatives were plenty, the number more than two hundred. However from the beginning of the Chien An era to now, a period of less than ten years, two-thirds of them died, seven-tenths from *shang han* (febrile disease). I pitied those who were ill and could not be cured. So I studied the medicine of the old classics and collected many prescriptions and compiled the book *Shang han tsu ping lun.*" Thus having witnessed the death of his relatives from fever, Chang, determined to learn, began collecting old prescriptions and finally completed his great work. The febrile disease mentioned was felt to be a plague, maybe what we now know as typhoid fever.

In reviewing and comparing the prefaces of the various editions of the *Shang han lun,* the one written in the Sung dynasty mentions the *Su wen* (Simple Questions), *Nan ching* (Difficult Passages in the *Nei ching),* *Yin yang ta lun* (Great Discourse on Yin and Yang), *Tai lu yao lu* (Herbal Compendium) and *Ping mai pien chen* (Pulse Palpation and Confirmation Discrimination). These works, however, are mentioned in the footnotes in the Kang Ping edition and so will be discussed elsewhere.

In the original text of the editions of the *Shang han lun* that we have nowadays, there is no evidence to imply that the *Shang han lun* had been influenced by the *Su wen* or the *Nan ching*. However, their influence is found in sections that were subsequently added to the *Shang han lun* by succeeding investigators.

Further discussion is warranted on the authorship of the preface and any clues that it may furnish us as to how the *Shang han lun* came to be.

The preface of the Sung edition of the *Shang han lun* is followed by the words, "By Chang Chi, Magistrate of Changsha, residing at Nan Yang, Han dynasty." Therefore, the preface would appear to have been written by Chang Chi. However, in the Kang Ping edition, there is no signature at the end of the preface; rather these words are located at the beginning of the text. This may have been due to editorial prerogative or possible carelessness on the part of the copier or typesetter with the text beginning immediately after the preface and this phrase inserted between the two sections. The placement of these words whether at the end of the preface or beginning of the text confuses the reader as to the identity of the author.

Keisetzu wrote a paper entitled "The Various Aspects Concerning the Study of the *Shang han lun*" wherein many opinions were proposed relating to the authorship of the preface. There are those who believe and others who disclaim that Chang Chung-ching wrote the preface. Some feel that the latter composed the first half and Wang Shu-ho the second half. These theories will be discussed further.

Evidence against the Theory that Chang Chung-ching Wrote the *Shang han lun*

Nakanishi Shinsai[7] states that scholars prior to the Chin-Han period did not write prefaces to their works. He further says that the sentence structure of the preface differs from that of the text which leads him to the conclusion that the preface was compiled by others. However, some investigators refute this theory. They feel that the *Shang han lun* was written in the period from the end of the Eastern Han to the Wei dynasties, so it is not appropriate to compare it with books composed before the Chin or Han dynasties. They believe also that Chang Chung-ching was the editor rather than the author of the volume. He merely collected references from previous medical treatises and well-known prescriptions, and this is why the preface and text differ in style. This point is well taken in determining the origin of the *Shang han lun*.

Toi Toiyori[8] feels that although the preface is attributed to Chang Chung-ching, the style of writing varies from that usually known to be Chang's. For instance, although the preface lists the *Su wen* and *Nan ching,* there were no further references to them in the text. Also, the preface refers to the biography of Pien Ch'iao from the *Shih chi* (Historical Records) which was not even written at the time of Chang Chung-ching. He suggests that the preface was written by another individual. Toiyori's reasoning is based on his assumption that the text of the *Shang han lun* was completed by Chang Chung-ching. Since the composition of the preface and text vary, and the references used in the former do not appear in the latter, he feels another author compiled the preface. Toiyori appears, however, to be in error regarding the Pien Ch'iao story. The *Shih chi* was originally known as *Tai shih kung su* and completed during the Western Han dynasty (206 B.C.-A.D. 24). The name was changed to *Shih chi* during the Wei-Tsin period ca. the third century A.D. Although the title was altered, the contents were unchanged. This means that Chang Chung-ching did have access to Pien Ch'iao's biography. Note: Chu Nan-hsi[9] and Yuan Yuan-lin[10] also believed that the preface was written by others.

Theory that Chang Chung-ching Composed the First Half of the Preface and Wang Shu-ho the Second.

In his book *Shang han kao* (An Investigation of the *Shang han lun*)[11], Yamada Seitsin states that the first half of the preface from the beginning to "si kuo pan yi" (would have acquired most of the knowledge) was written by Chang Chung-ching and from "fu tien pu wu hsing" (heaven has arranged the five elements) to the conclusion was composed by Wang Shu-ho. He gave the following evidence in support of his premise.

1. The phrase "si kuo pan yi" was a method used to conclude an essay, the part following it representing a different argument.
2. The first and second sections are of varying context and style.
3. The person called Yueh Hen in the first half is called Pien Ch'iao in the second half. Again here, this indicates that the work was not completed by one individual.
4. Some sentences in the first part are repeated in the second.
5. Chang Chung-ching never mentioned the five elements or the meridians, but these are included in the discussion in the second part.
6. Chang Chung-ching never gave information on the three locations or nine symptoms method of pulse diagnosis, nor did he include data regarding observations relative to the frontal and facial complexion procedures of diagnosis.
7. The expression "I pitied those who were ill and could not be cured" seems to be a proper closing to end the first section.

Seitsin's reasoning appears logical although points 5 and 6 are disputable. His suggestions as to different authorship of the two parts are important. Some also point out that in the Kang Ping edition of the *Shang han lun* the first half of the preface averaged fifteen words per line and the second thirteen; this also implies that the second portion was added later. Yito Osuke[12] agrees with Seitsin's conclusion.

Available Data Favoring Chang Chung-ching as the Author of the Preface.

Katakura Tsururio[13] is the main proponent of this school of thought agreeing with the opinion expressed by Wu Cheng (Yuan dynasty) in the preface of his work *Huo jen su pen*. They both feel that the preface of the *Shang han lun* was more of a compilation of all the previously available works on the subject and merely edited by Chang Chung-ching. This would easily explain the differences in style of the two parts and not contradict the authorship of Chang.

85

Some of the data available on the lost works of Chang Chung-ching allow the following conclusions. Chang inherited the traditions of medicine that prevailed in the Three Kingdoms and Six Dynasties period which were based on the system of the *Huang ti nei ching*. The system stressed the universal view of the five elements and the system of numbers, the celestial stems, the five "viscera" and the six "bowels", and the theory of the meridians. Viewed from this standpoint, it is still a possibility that the second half of the preface could have been written by Wang Shu-ho because, as Seitsin has pointed out, both Chang and Wang were distinguished proponents of the *Huang ti nei ching* system of medicine. However, a final conclusion in this respect is still difficult to arrive at in the absence of supporting evidence.

From the above discussion, it seems clear that the original text of the *Shang han lun* was written in a language form which antedated that commonly used in the Wei-Han period. Chang Chung-ching merely edited it and put in his own views while he was doing so. Then Wang Shu-ho added his personal view when he reedited it.

Some investigators conclude that the *Shang han lun* was compiled in the eighth or ninth year of the Chien An era because Chang Chung-ching states in the preface, "From the beginning of Chien An period to now, it is less than ten years." This may well be wrong in view of the phrase "to now". It could mean "From the beginning of the Chien An, in less than ten years, two-thirds of the whole clan were dead. Therefore, the time meant by "to now" which he said was in the period between the eighth and ninth year of the Chien An era may actually have been a long time afterward, particularly taking into consideration that he wrote down the information from memory at a later date. The Chien An period lasted twenty-four years. It was succeeded by the perishing of the Late Han dynasty and the rising of the era of the Three Kingdoms. Therefore, it is reasonable to assume that the *Shang han lun* could have been completed at the end of the Chien An epoch or even in the Three Kingdoms cycle or ca. A.D. 200. This would coincide with the research of Wang Ping that Chang Chung-ching was born in the period between the end of the Late Han dynasty and the beginning of the Wei Kingdom.

The Geographic Background of the *Shang han lun*

Some information on the completion and geographical background of the *Shang han lun* is given in the *Tung yang i hsueh shih* (History of Oriental Medical Science) written by Otsuka Keisetsu in 1941. If we assume that the writing of the preface was done by Chang Chung-ching and that the original text was completed by him during the Warring States Period, there is no problem even though the two vary in their style of phraseology and composition. Yet In *Yi hsin fang*[14] (Cure Heart Formulas) the recorded Chang Chung-ching's prescriptions differ in phraseology from those quoted in the *Shang han lun*. If the original text of the *Shang han lun* was written in the period of the Warring States,[15] it is not difficult to understand why the diagnostic and therapeutic methods differed so much from those practiced by Pien Ch'iao and Chun Yu Yi. It is apparent that they belong to two different areas.

The medicine typified in the *Huang ti nei ching* was felt to arise in the Yellow River area in North China. Contrariwise, the beginning of the doctrine on healing as exemplified by the *Shang han lun* was felt to originate in the district south of the Yangtze River. Some evidence in favor of this premise may be found in the *Huang ti nei ching — Su wen* under the title of "Yi fa fang yi lun" (Discussion on Strange Methods and Prescriptions) where it is stated that Chinese medicine is adapted to the variations in geography and climate: e.g., therapy in the East is carried out by means of a stone probe; poisons are used in the West; moxa in the North; and the "nine acupunctures" in the South.[16] Secondly, the herbs recorded in the *Shang han lun*, such as evodia and zanthoxylum, bear prefixes of abbreviated designations of places such as Wu and Shu which are located south of Yangtze River. Some investigators have also postulated that the author served as magistrate of Changsha. Further, in the T'ang dynasty, Sun Si-miao in his masterpiece *Chien chin yao fang* (Golden Precious Formula) commented, "The physicians in the area south of the Yangtze River keep Chang's prescriptions secret and do not let others know." The most commonly used herb in the *Shang han lun* is cinnamon which is indigenous to South China. This herb has been mixed with corn to produce a sacrificial wine since the Warring States Period. The *Su wen* also states that cinnamon is a

87

wood grown in the region south of the Yangtze and is the most important of all herbs. The evidence, therefore, is overwhelming that the *Shang han lun* represents a collection of all available medical data in the region south of the Yangtze River.[18]

The *Huang ti nei ching* represents a system of medicine intrinsic to North China, depending primarily on the use of acupuncture and moxibustion. Pien Ch'iao and Ch'un-yu I (Ts'ang Kung) were proponents of this order of science in the Shang Tung Province. Their methods of diagnosis and treatment sharply diverge from those outlined in the *Shang han lun*.

In fact the *Huang ti nei ching* and the *Shang han lun* represent the two classical medical systems widely used in early China.[19] The former is the classic on acupuncture and moxibustion, and the latter represents the epic on herbal medicine. Developed independently, both are indispensable. In time the two branches were amalgamated and evolved into a single, strong medical discipline — traditional Chinese medicine as we know it today.

Footnotes to Chapter Three

1. Gihaku Furuya says in his *Chen wen shang han lun fu sheng pien* 正文傷寒論復聖辨 (A Discussion on the Text of *Shang han lun*) that he believes that Chang Chi and Chung-ching were fictitious.

2. Chang Hsien is listed in the *Annals* of *Emperor Hsien* 獻帝記 in the section "History of the Eastern Han Dynasty" 後漢書

3. In the *Shang han lun cheng chieh* 傷寒論正解 (The Correct Interpretation of *Shang han lun)* by Chiukei Chiotani, Chung Ching and Hua To were said to be contemporaries but this cannot now be verified in current standard references. Chiotani feels that the magistrate of Changsha Prefecture was mistaken for Chang Chung-ching and that Chang Chi was the writer of the interpretations and footnotes of the book. Therefore, while Wang Shu-ho was compiling his work he mistook Chang Chi for Chungching.

4. *Journal of Society of Oriental Medicine in Japan.* 5, 1

日本東洋醫學會誌

5. Wang Ping, *Interpretations of the Su-wen* 素問答
Pao Ying era, T'ang dynasty, A.D. 762.

6. *Chinese Medicine and Chinese Drugs* 漢方與漢藥 3:1.
January 1935.

7. Nakanishi Shin-sai, *Shang han ming su chieh* 傷寒名數解
(Vol. I)

8. Toi Toyori:, *Shang han lun ku hsun kou yi* 傷寒論古訓
口義

9. Chu Nan-hsi, *Shang han wai chuan* 傷寒外傳

10. Yuan, Yuan-lin, *Shang han lun ching yi* 傷寒論精義

11. Yamada Seitsin, *Shang han kao* 傷寒考

12. Gitó Osuke, *Shang han lun chang yi ting pen* 傷寒論張義
定本

13. Katakura Tsururio, *Shang han chi wei* (傷寒啓微).

14. The *Yi hsin fang* (醫心方) was written in the Hei An
era in Japan and is the oldest medical treatise known in Japan. It
was completed in A.D. 984 and cites many quotations from
Chinese medical works compiled in the Sui and T'ang dynasties in
China. Among these, there are eleven places where it states "Chang
Chung-ching says. . . ." For example, "If one wants to treat the
various diseases, first one has to clean up the five solid and the six
luminal organs with herbal decoctions and to channel the different
meridians." As one can see, the style used and ideas expressed are
completely different from those appearing in the *Shang han lun*
and this holds true with all the quotations.

15. Huang-fu Mi (A.D. 215-286) in the preface of his book
Chia i ching 甲乙經 on acupuncture states that the *Shang han
lun* was based on the hypothesis of "Tang yi lun" 湯液論
(Theory of Herbal Decoctions) by Yi Yin 伊尹 , the prime
minister of the Yin dynasty. This was the consensus of opinion
throughout Japan. There is also a volume entitled *Shang han lun
yi chien pien* 傷寒論易簡辨 , the author of which is unknown,
in which there is a paragraph that says that the *Shang han lun*
was completed in the period of the Warring States and was based
on the *I ching* 易經 (Book of Changes) and had incorporated
Sun Tze's theory. The style and grammar of the two volumes are
quite comparable.

16. Stone probes were needles usually made from flint.
Poisons as used here refers to decocted medicines. Nine acupunc-

tures relates to the different needles employed in therapy.

17. When Sun Si Miao 孫思邈 was writing *Chien chin yao fang* 千金要方 , he was unable to refer to the *Shang han lun* as the physicians in the region south of the Yangtze River (Changsha District 長沙) would not divulge Chang Chung-ching's prescriptions. This story has been recorded in his completed work. It was not until he compiled his *Chien chin yi fang* 千金翼方 thirty years later that he was able to cite material from the *Shang han lun*.

18. *Fujida Chiokuhito* 藤田直人 (A Study on the History of the Negotiations between the East and the West.)

19. Ishihara Akira, *I hsueh shih kai sho* 醫學史概說 (A Summary of Medical History). Kogawa Teisan, *I hsueh chih li shih* 醫學之歷史 (The History of Medical Science). The Eastern Han dynasty as used in this text is also known as the Later Han dynasty.

Chapter Four
The Dissemination and Subsequent Editions
of the *Shang han lun*

Various Names of the *Shang han lun*

As pointed out in the second section of Chapter Three, the *Shih chi* (Historical Records) were referred to originally as *Tai shih kung shu* in the Han dynasty, the current designation being initiated in the Wei and Chin dynasties. Another similar case is the *Ling shu* which was initially called *Chiu chuan* (Nine Volumes) or *Chen ching* (Needle Classic). The same is true for *Shang han lun* which was first entitled *Pien shang han* (The Identification of Fever Diseases) or *Chang Chung-ching fang* (Chang Chung-ching Prescriptions). It was also called at one time *Wang Su-ho Chang Chung-ching fang* (Wang Su-ho's Chang Chung-ching Prescriptions). The origin of the name *Shang han tsu ping lung* (Essay on Febrile and Miscellaneous Diseases) is fully discussed in the *Tang shu yi wen chih* (A Collection of the Literature and Technology of the T'ang Dynasty).

On the question as to how many volumes comprise each work, the *Pien shang han* and *Shang han tsu ping lun* were composed of ten parts each, whereas the remaining books mentioned above contained fifteen volumes each. One naturally wonders if the contents of the ten and fifteen varieties were the same. In this respect, it was a common occurrence in earlier periods for works composed of ten volumes to be divided subsequently into fifteen, and it was simple to do. The preface of the Sung edition, however, states that there are sixteen sections in the *Shang han tsa ping lun.*

It is quite possible that the fifteen volumes comprising the *Chang Chung-ching fang* and the *Wang Su-ho Chang Chung-ching fang* might represent a combination of the *Shang han lun* and *Chin kuei yao lueh*. Some researchers in the T'ang dynasty incorporated the *Shang han lun* and *Chin kuei yao lueh* into one book under the title of *Chang Chung-ching shang han lun,* the name used by Wang Tao (A.D. 675-755 A.D.) in his *Wai tai mi yao* (Medical Secrets).[1] A study of Wang's treatise indicates that the citations used through Volume 18 were taken from the *Chin kuei yao lueh.* Therefore, since the sequence of the material presented by Wang differs from that of the modern *Chin kuei yao lueh,* it can be assumed that the *Shang han lun* he used as a source was probably composed of at least 18 volumes.

The literary scholar Wang Chu of the Sung dynasty found a book entitled *Chin kuei yu han yao lueh fang* among many old moldy volumes located in a storage room. It was composed of three volumes: *Pien shang han* (Identification of the Shang Han), *Lun tsa ping* (Discussions of Miscellaneous Diseases), and *Chu chu fang* (Citations of Prescriptions). There was also a section on the treatment of female diseases. Again it is evident that the number of books varied. There are works bearing the title of *Shang han lun* whose contents are those of the *Chin kuei yao lueh* and those termed *Chin kuei yu han yao lueh fang* that are found to be the *Shang han lun.* Some researchers have attributed the *Chin kuei yu han chin* to a writer in the T'ang dynasty, but since it is not similar to the current version of *Chin kuei yao lueh* it is probably a different edition of the *Shang han lun.*

From the above information, it is obvious that the number of volumes comprising the *Shang han lun* are not fixed and even the content has varied from the very beginning. The great number of editions of this work can be explained by the fact that the reviewers appended their interpretations to the book in an effort to make it more comprehensible to the reader.

The *Huang ti nei ching* was the primary system of medicine

used in the Wei and Chin periods. When the *Shang han lun* appeared, it represented an entirely different view of medicine; and, accordingly, Chang Chung-ching and Wang Su-ho incorporated into it some of the concepts originally from the *Nei ching* to make it easier for people to understand. This method, however, has made it more difficult for the modern scholar to analyze the two works.

"*Shang han tsu ping lun*" or "*Shang han tsa ping lun*"

As mentioned in the foregoing section, the work *Shang han lun* has been known under the various titles. However, the modern designation *Shang han lun* is an abbreviation of the full name *Shang han tsu ping lun*. The word *"tsu"* as used here has caused considerable controversy. Some think that it might have been mistaken for *"tsa"* (miscellaneous), a thought that has strong support. Taki Genkan,[4] noted for his meticulous research, agrees with this assumption. Other prominent scholars who share similar thoughts include Yamada Seisin,[5] Nori Kiyen,[6] Kitamura Tayeso,[7] and Yanagida Kowa.[8] However, as mentioned previously, the *Shang han lun* exists in two forms, one covering *shang han* and miscellaneous diseases and the other *shang han* alone. Lin I, et al. discovered a ten volume edition of the *Shang han lun* in the Sung dynasty and collated it. This became the prototype for the Sung edition of the *Shang han lun*. Yet for some unknown reason the title *Shang han tsu ping lun chi* was written before the preface. Only from the second line on did it say, "The *Lun* reads— — — —." So the word *"chi"* 集 (collective) in turn became a point of discussion. Yamada Seisin thinks that *"chi"* might represent the character *"hsu"* 序 meaning "preface". However, books bearing the name *Shang han tsu ping lun chi* existed prior to the Sung dynasty, and the same designation also appeared in the newly revised preface of the *Su wen*.[9] Hence the work found by Lin I, et al., probably was one of those which bore the word *"ch'i"*.

The Kang Ping edition of the *Shang han lun* uses the title *Shang han tsu ping lun* without the character *"chi"*. The first sentence of the preface "Each time I read the story of Chin Yueh-jen's travels to the State of Kuo— — —" was introduced with three characters meaning *"Chi Lun* said." Judging from this, it is pos-

93

sible that there is yet another book with the name *"Chi lun."* In the Sung edition, the character *"chi"* might have been placed a little farther away from the preface and closer to the title of the volume. The situation might appear as shown in the following: (The Kang Ping edition)

Shang han tsu ping lun Chi lun states: "Every time I read the story . . ."

└─ These three characters were originally appended as a side-note to the main line.

(The Sung edition)

Shang han tsu ping lun chi   Lun states: "Every time I read the story. . ."

It is a matter of record that the title *Shang han tsa ping lun* does not appear in the *Record of Classics and Books of the Sui Dynasty,* in the old and new *Record of Literature and Technology* of the *T'ang Dynasty,* or in *The History, Literature and Technology of the Sung Dynasty.* It is found only in the preface of the Sung edition of the *Shang han lun.* The Kang Ping edition also used the designation *Shang han tsu ping lun.*

As mentioned previously, the name *Shang han tsu ping lun* was in *The Record of Literature and Technology* of the T'ang dynasty. However, Taki Genkan felt that the character *"tsu"* was an aberrant form of *"tsa"* primarily because the former is meaningless. For this reason he cannot comprehend why it was used in this way.

Otsuka also was aware of this problem and made the following comment in his book *The History of Oriental Medical Science:* "According to the *New Record of the T'ang Dynasty,* the work was also named *Chang Chung-ching shang han tsu ping ling.* Here the characters *"tsu ping"* meant "acute diseases" and *"shang han,"* "febrile diseases." Next, the volume which combined the *Shang han lun* and *Chin kuei yao lueh* was called originally *Shang han tsa ping lun,* but the latter term did not appear until the preface to the Sung edition of the *Shang han lun* and *Chin kuei yao lueh* collated by Lin I, et al.

Generations later, Taki Genkan, Mori Tachisore et al. regarded the character *"tsu"* as having been written in error for

94

"*tsa.*" Otsuka however disagrees. Initially he felt that "*tsu ping*" referred to acute diseases only, but later he found that the *Chin kuei yao lueh* was comprised primarily of chronic conditions but included many acute illnesses. However, in 1962 (20 years later), Iyu Yamamoto Seichiro put forth the theory that the character "*tsu*" of "*tsu ping*" could be interpreted to mean "to lead," as in "the leading soldier". Carried further this means that the Marshal *Shang Han* (as head of diseases) leads a host of diseases: i.e. *tsu ping* could be interpreted as the conditions caused by *shang han.*

Todo Meipo in *A Study on the Etymology of Chinese Characters* gives the following explanation for the character *tsu* which appears to confirm Seichiro's theory: "The character *tsu* 卒 was used to denote soldiers, it had the same meaning as the character *shuai* in *"yin shui"* meaning "to take the lead," signifying to concentrate the soldiers and take the initiative. This can be likened to the expression "ten bundles in one string." When used as a verb, *tsu* means to conclude as in *"tsu yeh"* connoting graduation; it implies a conclusion of all the past. But when used as an adverb, it symbolizes the termination, end or finale."

In conclusion, *Shang han tsu ping lun* means a medical treatise composed of the diagnosis and treatment of various diseases that resemble several soldiers led in orderly manner by *shang han.* Originally, *tsa* 雜 , in *Shang han tsa ping lun,* meant miscellaneous diseases like random soldiers. Therefore, whether the book was entitled *Shang han tsu ping lun* or *Shang han tsa ping lun,* the meaning was basically the same. The character *tsu* became incomprehensible to subsequent generations and the *Chin kuei yao lueh* became known as the *Tsa ping lun.* The *Chin kuei yao lueh* includes not only miscellaneous diseases of a mild nature, but also the more serious conditions as found in the *Shang han.*

Subsequent Editions of the *Shang han lun*

The *Shang han lun* was compiled by Chang Chung-ching ca. A.D. 200. Approximately one hundred years later, Wang Su-ho of the West Tsin dynasty revised the text by collecting all known, as well as previously scattered and lost data, written by Chang into one edition. Several generations later Wang was severely criticized and called "Chang's Betrayer." But the fact remains: Chang's great contribution to medicine may well have been lost forever without Wang's new edition. So actually, Wang's work deserves great credit, and he, a just appraisal for his efforts and contributions. A native of Kao Ping in the southeast area of Shang Tung Province, Wang's original name was Hsi. He also wrote *Mo ching* (Book on the Pulse) and served with distinction as a royal physician in the West Tsin dynasty.

Governor Kao Chi-ching compiled an edition of the *Shang han lun* during the Kai Pao years, ca. A.D. 970, of Emperor Tai Tsu of the Sung dynasty and thereafter presented it to the emperor. This work has been lost. Following this, several scholars including Kao Pao-hen, Sun Chi, and Lin I were commissioned by Emperor Ying Tsun in the Sung period to revise the *Shang han lun*. Their work, published in the second year of Chi Ping (1065), was the original Sung edition. It, too, however, has disappeared. Later, Chao Kao-mei re-edited the Sung volume which was widely distributed in China and in Japan.

The *Annotated Shang han lun,* the oldest of all annotated editions, was written by Cheng Wu-chi who was born around the Chih Ping years (1064-1067) of the Sung dynasty at Liu She which was later occupied by the state Chin and became part of the latter's territory. So Cheng Wu-chi was a Chinian citizen. He came of a family of generations of physicians and was very clever, concise, and learned. His other works include *Shang han ming li lun* (A Treatise on the Elucidation of the *Shang han lun)* and *Fang lun* (A Discourse on Herbal Prescriptions).

Another edition compiled by Asano Genfu in three volumes appeared in the ninth year of the Kuansei era (1797). It was *The Collated Sung Edition of the Shang han lun.* The "General Notes" stated that this publication was based on the earliest known Sung edition of the *Shang han lun.* However, this was not true as it was actually from the revised Sung edition by Chao Kai-me, since the arrangement of the context varied considerably from the original, a fact that is explained in detail in the *Chung ching chuan shu* (A Complete Set of Chung Ching's Books). The revised edition was used in absence of the primary work. The resulting book then was based on the volumes edited by Chao Kai-mei and Cheng Wu-chi. In addition, there were many other so-called Sung editions of the *Shang han lun,* among which perhaps the one most recognized was the *New Collated Sung Edition of the Shang han lun*[11] published in the fifteenth year of the Tienpo era (1884) as a replica of the *Zon sei do yaku shitsu tei hon* which was compiled by Inaba Genki under the tutelage of his teacher Taki Genken. Genki used Taki Genkan's manuscript *Shang han lun chi yi* as the basis for his work. Otsuka states that although the book had a reputation of being reliable it was not a faithful rendition.

One of the most popular editions of the *Shang han lun* has been the small type version published in the fifth year of the Seitoku period (1715). It was completed by Kakawa Shutoku who used Cheng Wu chi's *Annotated Shang han lun* in preparing his work but deleted the annotations and the section on drug processing. Its acclaim has been attributed to its small size which made it easy to carry.

The oldest Sung edition known in Japan appeared in the eighth year of the Kuanbun era (1668). According to the "Foreword" written by Okatsuru Gentei, the book was reprinted from a manuscript of the original and annotated by Gentei's teacher, Tachihaku. The epigraph states: "Cheng Wu-chi's *Annotated Shang han lun* has spread throughout Japan and is much more popular than the Sung edition." Otsuka feels that the Kuanbun edition was a good work although Shibuko Chusai and Mori Tachisore in *Ching chie fang ku chih* (An Archaeological Research of Classics and Books)[10] reported to the contrary.

Both the *Annotated Shang han lun* by Cheng Wu-chi, and *Chung ching chuan shu,* which includes the former, were reprinted in Japan. It is doubtful if Cheng Wu-chi's revision was widely distributed before the eighth year of the Kuanbun period. Further, a punctuated and annotated *Shang han lun* was published in the fourth year of the Hiroka era (1847). This book collated all previous editions and was printed in the style of small type. The style used proved helpful to the reader in studying the work.

Taki Genkan tells about an edition called *Chin kuei yu han ching* which was known in the T'ang dynasty. It was collated by Kao Pao-hen, Sun Chi, Lin I, et al., in the third year of the Chih Ping era in the Sung dynasty. On its completion, the authors submitted an official report to the emperor stating, "Your royal subjects have reviewed and revised all the known medical works as your Majesty requested. First, the *Shang han lun* was studied, followed by the present research which differed in some aspects, but the completed volume is in compliance with the wisdom of

97

worthy predecessors, without basically altering the original text." Although reprinted in Japan, it was not as widely circulated as the Sung and Cheng editions.

Finally, Otsuka in modern times reviewed and compared many of the available, standard works on this subject, including the Kang Ping, Sung, Cheng, Yu-Han and other editions of the *Shang han lun*, and published his own study in 1937.

Review of the Kang Ping Edition of the *Shang han lun*

Otsuka purchased two transcribed volumes (upper and lower) of the Kang Ping edition of the *Shang han lun* in a book store at Hongkyo in Tokyo in the early autumn of 1936. One of the greatest differences between the Kang Ping edition and the Sung and Cheng revisions is the deletion of the two chapters *"Pien mo fa"* (Pulse Identification Methods) and *"Ping mo fa"* (Pulses in the Healthy Individual). Another difference is the composition which is rendered in lines averaging thirteen to fifteen characters with annotations interpolated in fine print throughout the text.

Using the Kang Ping, Sung, and Cheng's edition of the *Shang han lun*, another Kang Ping reprint and Waki's early version of the *Shang han lun*, Otsuka wrote an article entitled "The Kang Ping Edition of the *Shang han lun*" for the December 1936 issue of the *Journal of Chinese Medicine and Medicinals*. He discussed the similarities and differences of the various available works on the subject.

The following are a few points that may contribute to a greater understanding of the Kang Ping edition of the *Shang han lun*. This work was so named to distinguish it from the Sung and Cheng interpretations and from Waki's *Ancient Edition of the Shang han lun* which was well known in the Tokugawa era. The only volumes known in the Heian period (1058-1068) were the *Shang han lun* and the *Shang han tsu ping lun*. Kang Ping Corresponds to the Heian Period of Japan and was the period during which Tancha Gachu, Japan's "Pien Ch'iao", was most active. The book derived its name from the inscription "Gachu in the third year of Kang Ping." Waki's *Ancient Edition of the Shang han lun* received its name from a research article which Waki Shisei wrote on the subject following the format of the Kang Ping edition in the second year of the Teiwa Period (1346). The style had been known since the Kamakura era which indicates that the King Ping version was in existence at that time. Waki's is the only rendition that has maintained its original form in Japanese and has not been subjected to revisions.

One must be cautious in completely accepting the authenticity of the Kang Ping edition due to likely errors made during its numerous transcriptions over the years. However, in the text, the lines composed of fifteen words each are close to the original form. Additional changes were made by succeeding generations including annotations and interpolations.

Otsuka has discussed the similarities and differences between the Sung and Kang Ping editions elsewhere. He points out that in the first half of the preface from the beginning to the line "Then one may comprehend quite a lot" each line is composed of fifteen words, whereas in the text there are thirteen words to each line. (This is further discussed in his explanation of the preface.) There was no signature of the author in the Kang Ping edition, only two lines which appeared before the words "The Notes of *Shang Han*": "Written by Chang Chi, Magistrate of Changsha, residing at Nan Yang in the Han dynasty" and "Compiled by Wang Su-ho, Royal Physician in the Chin dynasty." Both lines preceded the text. The two chapters on "Pulse Diagnosis" and "Pulses in the Healthy Individual" were placed before the "Notes on the Shang han" in the Sung and Cheng editions but were not included in the Kang Ping rendition. The majority of previous Japanese researchers consider these two chapters to have been added by Wang Su-ho. However, Otsuka feels that they did not appear until the T'ang dynasty, because the chapter context on the pulse differed from Wang Su-ho's *Mo ching* (Pulse Classic). Even here, he is uncertain as he goes on to say that perhaps they could have been completed by Chang Chung-ching. Most researchers reasoned that the two chapters must have been composed by Wang Su-ho because the theory on the pulse was contradictory.[12] Otsuka feels that the first *Shang han lun* was not an original work written by Chang Chung-ching, but rather it represented a compilation of all prior materials available. This would account for the differences in pulse concepts.

Notwithstanding the above facts, Otsuka maintains that much of the *Shang han lun* was completed by Wang Shu-ho, giving as evidence material in Wang Tao's *Wai tai mi yao,* in which are cited frequent examples from the *Shang han lun* that are introduced by the words "Wang Su-ho said."[13] Correlating these examples with the principles, style of writing, and quotation "Now I have collected all of Chung-ching's ancient theories————" one has the feeling that the work is Wang Su-ho's. However, some of the thirteen word lines concerning the *Yung Chi Lun* (Phase movement theory) could have been written in the Sui-Tang period.

If one assumes that the Kang Ping edition of the *Shang han lun* was written by an early herbalist in the Tokugawa era, then the theory that the *Shang han lun* was written by Wang Su-ho would have to be eliminated.

There is a chapter entitled *Pien ching shih yeh mai chen* following "Notes on the *Shang han*" in both the Sung and Cheng editions of the *Shang han lun.* There is also a chapter called *Pien ching shih yeh* (Identification of Convulsions, Rheumatism, and Heat Stroke) in the *Yu han* edition. This latter subject was originally discussed in the *Chin kuei yao lueh* in which the conditions were described in greater detail together with representative prescriptions. The reason why this portion appeared in the *Shang han lun* can be answered by reviewing the Kang Ping edition. The latter has *Pien tai yang ping ching shih yeh* (Identifications of Convulsions, Rheumatism and Heat Stroke in the Greater Yang Diseases) with an explanatory note "caused by *shang han*" placed adjacent to the characters "tai yang ping" and another note "these three diseases are better discussed separately, but as they are similar to shang han, they are mentioned here" interpolated under the entry "Ching shih yeh". Therefore, briefly, the greater yang diseases caused by *shang han* are similar to *ching, shih, yeh.*

The *Chen-wu-tang* formula in the Sung and Cheng's editions and the *Yu Han* was called *Hsuan-wu-tang* in the Kang Ping version. The characters referred to the name of the God in charge of the North.[14] Hsuan was changed to Chen to avoid using the name of Emperor Hsuan Tsu of the Sung dynasty. Also *Szu-ni-tang* and *Szu-ni-san* used in the Sung work was changed to *Huei-ni-tang* and *Huei-ni-san* in the Kang Ping volume, because of an error in transcription. The correct character is *huei* 回 , meaning "to restore." In referring to the custom of designating prescriptions by their use, it is obvious that the word *szu* 四 is inappropriate. In that this represents a formula to cure that patient from *chieh ni* (coldness and exhaustion of the four limbs), it is more reasonable to name it *huei* (to restore) *ni tang*. Moreover, in the Kang Ping book, *Tai yang ping* was written as *Ta yang ping* and *Tai yin ping* as *Ta yin ping*. *Tai* and *Ta* are synonymous. Other minor differences will not be discussed at this time. Actually, all editions need to be carefully reviewed and compared.

Authenticity of the Kang Ping Edition

The Kang Ping edition is the definitive edition in that it preserves the classic style of the Chin dynasty. This opinion is shared by Tohen Heysan and Ishihara Akira. However, others such as Mizukumo Genkyu regarded it as a counterfeit edition. Otsuka Keisetsu wrote an article on "Recognition and Supplementation of the Kang Ping Edition of the *Shang han lun*"[1] which appeared in the October 1939 issue of *Kan po to kan yaku* (Chinese Medicine and Chinese Medicinals). He stated:

> "The book I got this time was Waki's *Ancient Edition of the Shang han lun* composed of the upper and lower volumes. In another article on the "Chronological Changes of the Kang Ping Edition of *Shang han lun*" I have said that Waki's *Ancient Edition of the Shang han lun* has the same contents as the Kang Ping edition. But the book carried hand written legends by Iue Keiyen, who went under the sobriquet *Shien Tai I Shih* (Medical Practitioner of the Divine Platform), and Mizukumo Genyu. Keiyen wrote his words in the first year of Ansei and said he obtained the book from the proprietor of Kauseito Clinic whom he had known for years. However, the existence of Kauseito Clinic is debatable and remains a problem pending further research and verification. Genkyu's legend was written in the first year of Banyen and talks of his involvement in the collation of an offset copy owned by Saitaki. The corrections were done in red with the Chinese brush. The relationship between Mizukumo Genkyu and Iue Keiyen is not clear. But it is known that six years after Keiyen wrote in the book, he rejoined Saitaki's collation effort and corrected the errors in transcriptions. From these facts we know that the book was a scarce item in that time and was also transcribed by incompetents. There are other offset editions in existence."

101

After Otsuka Keisetsu wrote the above article, he found another Waki's *Ancient Edition of the Shang han lun,* complete in one volume, carrying the same preface by Iue Keiyen and a legend by Mizukumo Genkyu. In this edition, Genkyu wrote in red ink the following:

> The third year of Kang Ping was equivalent to the fifth year of Chia Yuo during the reign of Emperor Jen Tsun of the Sung dynasty of China. This was years before Lin I et al. did their collation. Thus this edition might represent the former classical style characteristic of the Han and Chin dynasties. However, the footnotes and sidenotes are mainly in compliance with the theories of more modern herbalists. This arouses suspicion that the edition was a phony. My friend I Non Ei has said, "No ancient transcriptions from Chinese Imperial regimes ever went without punctuation and phonetics and these are absent in this edition. This gives credence to the belief that it is an ancient edition."

The two reasons cited by Genkyu for believing the book to be spurious are: the differences in the linguistics of classical and non-classical literatures and the assumptions of herbalists in the Tokugawa era. Both points are doubtful because after reading the explanations of the various physicians after Nakanishi Shinsai's time, one finds out that the diagnostic methods outlined in the Kang Ping edition of the *Shang han lun* do not differ and the punctuation and phonetics could have been inadvertently or carelessly omitted by the transcriber.

It is said that a badly damaged copy of this book is in existence to which is attached the punctuation system of "Fu Ku Chi Tien" (the four corners of the Chinese characters are marked with specific symbols to facilitate reading) characteristic of the early years of the Kamakura era. If this copy could be found, the suspicions of Genkyu et al. would be cleared.

Footnotes

1. *The Wai tai mi yao* 外臺秘要 in four volumes was completed by Wang Tao in A.D. 752 while he was working in the Royal Library.

2. Kao Pao-hen, Sun Chi and Lin I in their preface to the

Chin kuei yao lueh fang 金匱要略方 written in the Sung dynasty indicate that the *Chang Chung-ching shang han tsa ping lun* 張仲景 傷寒雜病論 comprised sixteen volumes, but recent editions of the *Shang han lun* have appeared in ten volumes. The words "Tsa Ping" are either missing or abridged in various herbalist prescription books. Wang Chu discovered the three volumes of Chung Ching's *Chin kuei yu han yao lueh fang* 金匱玉函要略方 during his service in the Royal Library.

3. Taki Genkan states in the "General Notes" for the *Shang han lun chi yi* 傷寒論輯義 that the *Chin kuei yu han ching* 金匱玉函經 is a different edition of the *Shang han lun* with the same context but another title, and that it was written sometime before the T'ang dynasty. Its contents also seemed quite similar to that cited in the *Chien chin yi* 千金翼.

4. Taki Genkan, *Shang han lun chi yi tz tsuon kai* 傷寒論輯義之綜槪 (A Summary of the Definitions of *Shang han lun*).

5. Yamada Seisin in *Shang han lun chi chen* 傷寒論集成 said that the previous transcribers of the early editions mistook the character *tsu* for *tsa*, and this error was transmitted through subsequent revisions.

6. Mori Kiyen (Tachisore), *Shang han lun kao chu* 傷寒論考註 (The Research and Annotation on the *Shang han lun).*

7. Kitamura Tayeso commented on this problem thusly in his commentary *Shang han lun shu yi* 傷寒論疏義 , *"Tsu ping* has been mistaken for *tsa ping."* Kuo Yuon stated, *"Chung ching hsu lun* 仲景敍論 indicates that the *Shang han tsa pin lun* 傷寒雜病論 is composed of sixteen volumes."* Tayeso said that this represented an error in transcription, with the translator often omitting the radical or a character with too many strokes or combining two characters into one. Therefore, *tsa* was written with just the left radical or even as *tsu* alone.

8. Yanagida Kowa, *The Inductive Interpretation of the Shang han lun* 傷寒論繹解

9. In the beginning of Volume I of *The Re-expanded, Re-supplemented and Re-annotated Huang Ti's Nei Ching and Su Wen* 重廣補記黃帝內經素問 one reads that according to research Wang did not know the meaning or reason why the *Su wen* was so named or in what dynasty it was first used. Investigation has revealed that it initially appeared in *The History, Classics,*

103

Literatures, and Records of the Sui Dynasty 隋書經籍志 ·
In the Chin dynasty, Huang-fu Mi (A.D. 215-286) wrote in the
preface of his *Chia i ching* 甲乙經 that the *Su wen* 素問 discussed the various diseases in a very precise and discriminative
manner. Wang Su-ho (A.D. 210-285) of the Western Chin dynasty
said in *Mai ching* (Pulse Classic) that the science of the pulse was
derived from the *Chen ching* 鍼經 (Needle Classic) found in the
Su wen. Chang Chung-ching stated his book *Shang han tsu ping
lun chi* was based on the *Su wen.* From this evidence, then it is
fairly certain that the *Su wen* had appeared as early as *The
Historic Record of the Sui Dynasty* 隋志 in the Han era. There
were no records of this type available before Chang Chung-ching's
time. Later works also refer to the fact that the *Su wen* was
known in the Han dynasty. The above dates indicate that the
Shang han lun, as well as the preface, was written in the Han
dynasty. Further data relative to the origin of the *Su wen* is
needed, however, to make a definite conclusion.

    10. *Ching chi fang ku tz* 經籍訪古志 — Volume 7.
This book states that although the Kuanbun edition is still in
print, it is not entirely satisfactory and resembles the Sung reprint.
Its circulation continues to decrease.

    11. The "General Notes" from *The New Collated Sung
Edition of the Shang han lun* 新校宋板傷寒論 state that
Chao's edition of the *Shang hun lun* is similar to the Sung version
and the best book available of this type. However, it is heavy and
cumbersome for the student to carry. Fortunately, subsequent
condensations and abridgements of such things as annotations by
previous authors, particularly in the Sung period, have solved the
problem. Another edition compiled from Chao's work is Lekiyin's
Shang han lun chi yi 傷寒論輯義 .

    12. Taki Genkan in his *Shang han lun chi yi* 傷寒論輯義
states that the three chapters "Pien mo fa", "Ping mo fa" and
"Shang han li" were compiled by Wang Shu-ho who reviewed and
commented on available resources. They occasionally include
some of Chang Chung-ching's theories, but they actually differ
from the 397 rules."

    13. Wang Tao in his *Wai tai mi yao* quoted from "General
Notes for the *Shang han*" the following lines: "The *shang han*
diseases vary from day to day in severity" down to "It is suitable
to diagnose twice"; and the lines from "Thriving Yang and weak

Yin" down to "is not that very heartbroken." quoted in *Wai tai mi yao* and *Chien chin yao fang* to be words belonging to 'Wang Su-ho states' ".

14. In his *Shang han kao* 傷寒考 (A Research on the *Shang han lun)* Yamada Seishan said, "In ancient times, using the names of the Four Gods for designating prescriptions was not done for any particular reason. Some of the explanations given were that *Ching lung* (blue dragon) was used because *ma-huang* (Ephedrae Herba) was green or bluish in color; *Pai hu* (white tiger) was used because of the whiteness of gypsum; *Chu chueh* (red sparrow), because of the redness of zizyphus; and *Chen wu,* (a god of the North whose face is black), because of the blackness of aconite. People of subsequent generations associated this with the theory of the Five Elements and attached profound significance to the names. This is misleading. For if *ching lung* suggests dispersion, then does *pai hu* mean astringency? Or if *pai hu* implies a cool, cleaning agent, then does *chen wu* symbolize a strong, cold substance? Such correlations are quite impractical.

Otsuka found the following information about the use of the Four Gods' names. The chapter "Chu Li" 曲禮 (Etiquette of Music) in the *Li Chi* 禮記 (Records of Rites) says: "When marching, *Chu chueh* (朱雀) is in the front; *Hsuan wu* (玄武) (or *Chen wu)* in the rear; *Ching lung* (靑龍) to the left and *Pai hu* (白虎) to the right." In Kon Ying-ta's volume it says, *Chu chueh, Hsuan Wu, Ching lung* and *Pai hu* are the names of the celestial stars located at the four corners. *Hsuan wu* is the turtle with a protective shell to ward off attack". Chen Hau says, "Marching refers to the troops, whose banners are designated as *Chu chueh, Ching lung, Pai hu,* and *Hsuan wu* signifying the celestial stars at the four corners." The *Wu tsa tsu* records, "Chen wu is the same as *Hsuan wu* and is the god of one of the four corner stars; the others being *Chu chueh, Ching lung,* and *Pai hu.* The name *Chen wu* was substituted to avoid use of *Hsuan wu* which was the name of one of the Sung emperors." This is confirmed in the *Wan wei yu lun* 宛委餘論 where it reads, *"Hsuan wu* was changed to *Chen wu* to refrain from using the name of Emperor Hsuan Tsu of the Sung dynasty." Naito Konan commented in the section on the Sung and Yuan editions in his work *A Study of Oriental History* 東洋文化史研究 "To abstain from employing the *huei* (deceased emperor's name) of the emperor does not mean to eschew using the appellation of the ruling emperor."

15. *Chung wai i shih hsin pao* 中外醫事新報 (Medical News, Domestic and Foreign), No. 1245.

16. *Han fang chih lin chuang* (Practical-Kampo) Volume 9, No. 10. 漢方之臨床

Chapter Five
Research Trends
on the *Shang han lun* in Japan

Restoration of Traditional Chinese Medicine

When Confucianism replaced Buddhism in the ruling class in the Tokugawa kingdom, the mental attitude of feudal society was greatly influenced. During this period the field of medicine was led by Manase Dosan who incorporated into it Lee's and Chu's religious meditations as well as the many advancements in knowledge of the Sung age. The main concepts were the perennial opposites yin and yang, *wu hsing* or the five elements and the *ching-lo* (the longitudinal and latitudinal meridians). Medicine became more standardized in the Chin-Yuan dynasties.

Itso Jinsai advocated time-honored learning as opposed to the developments in the Sung period. Nagoya Genyi (1625-1696) initially studied only Lee's and Chu's works, but on reviewing *Shang han shang lun* (Exposition on the *Shang han lun*) and *I men fa lu* (Medical Rules), he gradually abandoned these old concepts; and, although not always sound in his ideas, recommended restoration of Chang Chung-ching's philosophy.

After the death of Genyi, the traditional school of thought under the tutelage of Goto Gonsan, Kakawa Shutoku, Matsuhara Ikansai, Sankyo Toyo, and Yoshimasu Todo further stressed the teachings of the *Shang han lun*. Referred to as the Ancient

Prescription School, it gradually replaced Lee's and Chu's methods, the Late Generation School, in the dawning of Japanese herbal medicine. This dualistic methodology never existed in China as it did in Japan.

The revival and popularity of the Ancient Prescription School was largely due to the efforts of Ito Jinsai and Gisei Sorai. Their predecessors in the Tokugawa era were also influenced by the Ancient Prescription School. Kakawa Shutoku under the tutelage of Ito Jinsai studied the classics and developed his theory of the "Unification of Confucianism and Medicine". Sorai's influence was felt through his disciple Yamaken Shunan (who corresponded with Sankyo Toyo and Taki Tsurutai) and Shunan's students Taki Tsurutai and Yoshimasu Todo. Todo, recognizing the ability of one of Toyo's students, Nagatome Kokushuan, felt threatened and said, "This man will certainly succeed me as the Doyen (dean) of Japanese medicine after my death." The above interest in the ancient school was reflected in an increased interest in study and research of the *Shang han lun* beginning ca. 1600.

The first annotations on the *Shang han lun* in China were completed by Cheng Wu-chi who was stimulated by the more general acceptance of *Huang Ti nei ching - Su wen* and *Ling shu.* He introduced *ching-lo* (longitudinal and latitudinal meridians) and the *Nei ching's* concept into his work. The Japanese readily accepted the opinions of these Chinese scholars about the *Shang han lun.* However, the herbalists of the Ancient Prescription School and their students believed that the philosophy of the *Shang han lun* and the *Nei ching* were widely divergent, and that one could not readily adapt the *ching-lo* concept into the *Shang han lun* system of medicine. These practitioners, therefore, de-emphasized the *Nei ching* in favor of their own school of thought. However, most doctors continued to incorporate and juggle both concepts in their work. Often, this led to disclaiming the *Shang han lun* when attempting to discuss and relate it to the *Nei ching.* Confusion also resulted from the *Shang han lun* proponents' worldly point of view in their interpretation of the original, as well as the many commentaries added by subsequent investigators. Sorai did much to clarify this situation.

Although the *Nei ching* was highly respected and never

108

seriously questioned from early times, it came in doubt with the advent of the Ancient Prescription School. In fact, Yoshimasu Todo of this group entirely denied the five element and yin-yang theories. (These concepts had developed independently but were closely associated with the *Nei ching*.)

According to the five element theory as applied to medicine, disease was felt to be a result of an imbalance among the five elements: wood, fire, earth, metal and water. Restoration of harmony was regarded as vital to treatment. The *ching-lo* circulation theory propounded that there was a pathway of energy— any disorder of which resulted in illness and the correction of which would result in cure. The herbalists of the ancient prescription group regarded these theories as superstitious and illogical. Sankyo Toyo said that he had studied the *Ling shu* and *Su wen* from childhood and never found them to be helpful.[1] Todo also regarded the work as spurious[2] and felt it was completed before the Chin dynasty. Japanese scholars came to emphasize the importance of research on the *Shang han lun* alone rather than attempting to mesh it with the concepts of the *Nei ching*.

Annotated Editions of the *Shang han lun*

Takino Kazuo reviewed Japanese editions in an article entitled "A Bibliography of Books on the *Shang han lun*" which appeared in the *Journal of the Oriental Medical Society of Japan*. Five hundred and thirteen different editions were listed, but the actual figure in existence may well be higher.

Otsuka catalogued forty of the more outstanding works of the above, some of which are in his personal library. (Those published after 1926. during the Showa era are exceptions.) These books are:

1.   a.   *Shang han lun pien cheng* 傷寒論辨正 (Identification and Verification of the *Shang han lun*) was written by Nakanish Shinsai and is composed of three volumes divided into six sections. The book starts with "Pien tai yang ping mo cheng ping chih fa shang" 辨太陽病脈證并治法上(The First Part: Identification of Greater Yang Diseases, Their Pulses, Con-

firmations, and Treatment) and concludes with "Pien yin yang i cha hou lau fu ping mo cheng ping chih fa" 辨陰陽易差後勞復病脈證并治法 (Identification of Diseases Attributed to Relapse and Recurrent Diseases due to Exhaustion after Recovery). Each section is accompanied by Shinsai's explanatory notes and unique views. This work, written in Chinese, represents a very creative undertaking. It attained a wide circulation at one time. The main text of the *Shang han lun* is separated from the comments and annotations added by other individuals.

b. *Shang han ming shu chieh* 傷寒名數解 (Various Interpretations of the Name *Shang han*) was also authored by Nakanish Shinsai and consists of five volumes in five sections. It, too, is in Chinese and covers the following subjects: *san yin, san yang,* (the three yin's and the three yang's); *shang han chung feng* (severe cold and wind stroke or apoplexy); and *ho ping* and *ping ping* (combinations or complications of disease). These two books can be regarded as the latitute and longitude of the study of the *Shang han lun*.

2. *Shang han lun chi cheng* 傷寒論集成 (A Collective Work on the *Shang han lun*) was compiled by Yamada Seishin and comprises ten volumes. Annotations are included in the preface along with interpretations for the various parts from "The First Part in the Identification of Greater Yang Diseases, Their Pulses, Confirmation and Treatment" down to "Identification of Diseases Attributed to Relapse and Recurrent Diseases Due to Exhaustion after Recovery." This book differs from *Shang han lun pien cheng* in that it quotes the theories of many distinguished Chinese and Japanese progenitors, and it distinguishes the context˜ from the annotations.

Seishin also completed another volume in research on the *Shang han lun* entitled *Shang han kao* 傷寒考 (A Research on the *Shang han lun*). This revealed much new data on the subject. Both books are in Chinese.

110

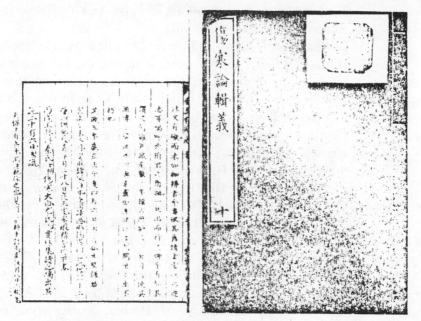

The *Shang han lun chi i* in which Taki Genken and Inaba Genki had written a lot of annotations

3. *Shang han lun chi i* 傷寒論輯義 (A Compendium on the Meaning of the *Shang han lun*) was written by Taki Genkan in ten volumes. The author relied on the opinion of noted Chinese scholars for his explanatory notes from "*Pien tai yang ping mai cheng ping chih fa shang*" to "*Pien yin yang i cha hou lau fu ping mai cheng ping chih fa*", rather than expressing his own opinions. The work is authentic and reliable and is widely read. It, too, is in Chinese.

4. *Shang han lun shu i* 傷寒論述義 (Explanatory Meanings of the *Shang han lun*) written also by Taki Genkan is in five volumes. A supplementary "Addendum to the Explanatory Meanings of the *Shang han lun*" was excluded in some editions. It is quite comprehensive and well thought out. It is in Chinese.

5. a. *Shang han lun fen chu* 傷寒論分註 (Partial Commentary on the *Shang han lun*).

111

b. *Shang han wai chuan* 傷寒外傳 (Extra Historical Record of the *Shang han lun*).

Both are in Chinese and were compiled by Tachibana Haruki. He made brief commentaries on the original text in the first work; the second consists of three volumes, the third of which adds little information.

6.　a.　*Ku hsun i chuan* 古訓醫傳 (Ancestral Doctrines Relating to Medicine) is a twenty-five chapter research written by Wutsuki Kontai. It is divided into four major parts: 1) "*I hsueh ching wu*" 醫學警悟 , a comprehensive explanation of the *Shang han lun* and *Chin kuei yao lueh*; 2) "The Upper Chapter on the Wind, Chill and Fever Diseases" 風寒熱病方經篇 , an explanation of the *Shang han lun*; 3) "The Lower Chapter on the Wind, Chill and Fever Diseases" 風寒熱病方緯篇 , a critique on the *Chin kuei yao lueh*; and 4) "*Yao neng fang fa pien*" 藥能方法辨 (Instructions on the Efficiency of Herbs), a discussion of the reliability of each herb. The entire book is based on the *ch'i, hsieh* and *shui* (air, blood and water) theory.

7.　*Shang han lun i chieh* 傷寒論繹解 (Inductive Explanation of the *Shang han lun*) is a research in Chinese in ten volumes compiled by Enagida Kasai. It includes a preface with explanatory notes on three chapters—"*Pien mai fa*" (Pulse Identification), "*Ping mai fa*" (Pulses in a Healthy Individual); and "*Shang han li*" (Cases of Shang Han Disease). These chapters have been omitted in most other works of this type, since most books start with the "Identification of Greater Yang Diseases". Further, Kansai's book is extensively annotated throughout. It has become quite rare.

8.　a.　*Shang han lun shu i* 傷寒論疏義 (Exploration of the *Shang han lun* to Determine Its Meaning).

b.　*Shang han lun cha chi* 傷寒論劄記 (*Shang han lun*: Questions and Answers).

c.　*Ching fang chuan liang lueh shuo* 經方權量略說 (A Brief Discussion of Classical Formulas and Their Units of Measure).

112

These were all written in Chinese by Kitamura Taeso. The *Shang han lun shu i* is seven volumes. There is a commentary on the preface but the chapters on "Pulse Identification", "Pulses in a Healthy Individual", "Cases of Shang Han Disease", and "The Diseases of Spasm, Moisture (Rheumatism) and Heat Stroke" are omitted.

The *Shang han lun cha chi* and *Ching fang chuan liang lueh shuo* are each one volume. The former deals with research on questionable words, phrases, clauses, and sentences in the *Shang han lun* whereas the latter investigates the units of measure in the formulas of the *Shang han lun*.

9.   a.   *I ching chieh huo lun* 醫經解惑論 (Answers to the Puzzles in the Medical Classics).

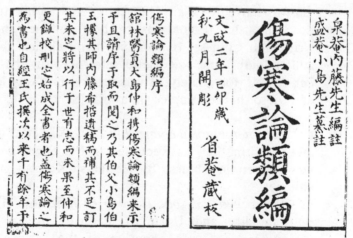

The foreword of *Shang han lun lei pien*

b.   *Shang han tsa ping lun lei pien* 傷寒雜病論類編(A Categorized Compilation of the *Shang han lun*).

The *I ching chieh huo lun* by Naito Kitetsu is three volumes totaling six sections. Kitetsu regarded the

Shen nung pen tsao ching (Shen Nung's Herbal Classic); *Huang ti ming tang ching* 黃帝明堂經 (Yellow Emperor's Classic); *Nei ching* 內經 (Classic of the Interior); *Pien Ch'iao nan ching* 扁鵲難經 (Pien Chiao's Classic on Medical Difficulties); and *Chung ching chin kuei yu han ching* 仲景金匱玉函經 (Chang Chung-ching's Synopsis of the Golden Chamber) as the five great classics of Chinese medicine—all are based on a similar point of view. He ingeniously introduced the concepts from the *Huang ti nei ching* and *Nan ching* into his *I ching chieh huo lun*. He also interpreted the *Shang han lun* in the light of the philosophy of the *Ju men shih chin* 儒門事親 (Attending the Parents as a Confucian Disciple) which included information on the viscera (solid and hollow) and *ching-lo*. Naito in this manner undertook the task of combining the *Nei ching* and *Shang han lun*, which resulted in many clinically provocative opinions.

The *Shang han tsa ping lun lei pien* 傷寒雜病論類編 was started by Naito but completed by his students posthumously. It contains thirteen volumes and was written in Chinese. It contains many clinical features and opinions that are useful references on the *Shang han lun*. Unfortunately, it was printed in a very limited edition so that few copies are available.

10. a. *Shang han lun mai cheng shih* 傷寒論脈證式(Pulses and Confirmations as Recorded in the *Shang han lun*) was written in Chinese by Kawaetsu Koozan in eight volumes.

b. *Shang han yao pin ti yung* 傷寒藥品體用 (The Substantiality and Usage of Medicine in the *Shang han lun*) describes the action of the various herbs in accordance with their use. The author seemed more interested in displaying his knowledge than contributing anything really worth while to the field.

11. *Shang han lun liu shih chuan* 傷寒論劉氏傳 (Liu's *Shang han lun*) in Chinese was done by Hakumizu Tahayoshi. It is composed of four volumes divided into

114

385 sections of which the first 268 comprise the main text with the remaining 117 consisting of addenda by investigators of subsequent generations. Annotations were made only on the main text. Tanayoshi was of the opinion that the first 268 sections had been completed by Pien Ch'iao Tsang et al. after the Warring States Period while the remainder was added by Wang Su-ho of the Chin dynasty and various scholars of the T'ang and Sung dynasties.

12. *Shang han lun te chieh* 傷寒論特解 (A Specific Interpretation of the *Shang han lun*) in Chinese was started by Saiseisai, continued by his student Hanai Moichi after his death, and finally completed by another disciple Asano Genfu after the death of Moichi. It has ten volumes. The 120 discussed sections of the *Shang han lun* are greatly detailed and at times redundant. Supplementary data from subsequent generations is appended.

13. *Shang han lun kuo tzu pien* 傷寒論國字辨(A Japanese Annotation of the *Shang han lun*) is a copy of the *Shang han lun te chieh* in eleven volumes. The main text is separated from the addenda and annotated in simple Japanese. This is suitable for the beginner.

14. *Shang han lun kuo tzu chieh* 傷寒論國字解 (A Japanese Explanation of the *Shang han lun*) was completed by Wunlinyin Ryosaku and is also intended for the neophyte. Simple notes are used and Japanese phonetic symbols are attached to the more difficult Chinese characters to aid pronunciation.

15. *Shang han lun ku hsun chuan* 傷寒論古訓傳 (Ancient Instructions in the *Shang han lun*). This research in Chinese in five volumes was completed by Kyusen Totani, allegedly according to the will of Yoshimasu Todo. However, it is contrary to Todo's known medical doctrine, and it is possible that Totani merely wished to gain recognition by using Todo's name. Notwithstanding, it does contain some noteworthy opinions.

115

16. *Shang han lun shih i* 傷寒論實義 (The True Meaning of the *Shang han lun*), a rare book in Chinese in five volumes, was written by Sousen Soan. Otsuka's copy originally belonged to Oda Kenzo, and another one is in the Congressional Library at Washington D.C. Soan believed that the ascending and descending principles of yin and yang were part of the *Shang han lun* and that any delection of this concept had been done by subsequent researchers. He then accordingly separated the *Shang han lun* into a primary text and a spurious text.

17. *Shang han lun tung tuan* 傷寒論通斷 (General Conclusions on the *Shang han lun*) is an excellent and enthusiastic work in Chinese compiled in ten volumes by Tokai Lintaimei. It is primarily a critique on *Shang han lun chi cheng* by Yamada Seishin and *Shang han lun pien cheng* by Nakanishi Shinsai.

18. *Shang han lun fang fa so pien* 傷寒論方法瑣辨 (A Detailed Study of the Prescriptions in *Shang han lun*) is a treatise composed of three volumes by Okada Seigo, a pupil of Yoshimasu Nangai. Among the latter's publications *Shang han lun ching i* and *Shang han lun cheng i* were based upon manuscripts completed by his disciples. However, Seigo's work is original and is an explanation of the *Shang han lun* based on the theories of *ch'i*, water, and blood.

19. *Shang han lun ching i wai chuan* 傷寒論精義外傳 (Extra-Historical Records on the Meaning of the *Shang han lun*) is a well-written, illustrated book by Wada Genyou, a pupil of Yoshimasu Nangai, who compiled the book to spread the doctrine of his master.

20. *Shang han lun cheng wen fu sheng chieh* 傷寒論正文復聖解 (A Review of the *Shang han lun* in Order to Restore the Master's Concepts) at times is difficult to comprehend. It was compiled by Furyua Shihaku who explained the *Shang han lun* according to the

116

theory of the "Changes". This is more adequately done than a similar work on this same point of view by Kinko Keisan: *Shang han lun shui huo chiao i kuo tzu pien.*

21. *Shang han lun cheng wen chieh* 傷寒論正文解 (Explanation of the Main Text of the *Shang han lun*) was written in eight volumes by Wada Toka. The explanation is concise and based upon clinical practice. All complicated research and reviews are omitted.

22. *Shang han lun yeh hua* 傷寒論夜話 (A Brief Report on the *Shang han lun*) is a review by Gen Nanyo consisting of four volumes. It includes commentary only up to the section on lesser yang disease.

23. *Shang han lun chang i ting pen kuo tso pien* 傷寒論張義定本國字辨 (The Exposition of the *Shang han lun* 傷寒論張義定本) is Ito Osuke's investigation into the Upper and Lower Volumes of the *Shang han lun.* In Japanese, it goes as far as the part on greater yang disease.

24. *Shang han lun chueh i* 傷寒論闕疑 (Answers to Questions in the *Shang han lun*) is an eight volume review by Furuhayash Mimomo concerned only with explaining the *Shang han lun* rather than what is implied by the title of the book.

25. a. *Shang han lun ching i* 傷寒論精義 (The Essential Meaning of the *Shang han lun*) is five volumes by Gen Genlin in Chinese. It is confined to a discussion on the meaning of the *Shang han lun* from the personal experience and study of the writer. Annotations and references from other authors are not included.

b. *Shang han lun tu shuo* 傷寒論圖說 (Illustrations of the *Shang han lun*) explains the meaning of the *Shang han lun* through illustrations.

26. a. *Shang han lun cheng chieh* 傷寒論正解 (Correct Annotations from the *Shang han lun*) was completed by Chuke Chotani. It consists of eight volumes bound into two books and includes illustrations and an appendix. It is regarded as a bold innovation that brilliantly reviews the contributions of the sages of three early generations: Huang Ti, Shen Nung, and Fu Shi. In the General Notes, Chotani states he used the words *"cheng chieh"* because he wished to rectify inaccuracies and annotations on previous *Shang han luns* according to the "The Changes" of the Chou dynasty. He was not biased by the opinions of other annotators nor did he pick up tenets from the ancient physicians. Chotani recognized that his work might seem strage in view of the innovations in medical science in the T'ang and Sung dynasties but was not concerned. b. *Cheng fa ke lueh pu* 證法格略譜 (A Simplified Table of Confirmations and Remedies) also by Chotani who tabulated the various confirmations and prescriptions of *shang han* (fevers); *chung feng* (apoplexy), and san ying-san yang (diseases of the three yin and the three yang).

27. *Shang han lun ku hsun kou i* 傷寒論古訓口義 (Lectures on the Ancient Doctrine of the *Shang han lun*) was authored by Toi Toan and comprises eight volumes. Regarded as a bold innovation, some of the information is not entirely reliable.

28. *Chia ke shang han lun* 家刻傷寒論 (A Personal Interpretation of the *Shang han lun*) is an eight volume endeavor in Chinese by Hirooka Shicho. It contains no alterations as made by Chotani and Toan. Notwithstanding, it has good basic material, identifying the main text with appropriate annotations.

29. *Fu ku shang han lun cheng* 復古傷寒論徵 (A Verification of the Early *Shang han lun*) is a research completed by Tien Taigaku, a disciple of Saiseisai. It is a combination of two related books: the early *Shang han lun*

in one volume and a verification of the early *Shang han lun* in six volumes. The entire set is a portion of the *Shang han lun te chieh* (A Specific Interpretation of the *Shang han lun*).

30. *Shang han lun chang chu* 傷寒論章句 (Chapters and Sentences of the *Shang han lun*) in one volume by Yoshimasu Nangai was compiled by selecting chapters and sentences from the *Shang han lun* and arranging them in logical order under appropriate categories.

31. *Hsiu cheng shang han lun chuan lun* 修正傷寒論全論 (A Revision of the Complete Theory on the *Shang han lun*) in four volumes by Nakagawa Shiutei was written in a style similar to that used in Nangai's *Shang han lun chang chu.* The second and third volumes concern verification and the last is a collection of prescriptions recorded in the *Shang han lun.* Shiutei also published another book entitled *Shang han chuan lun* 傷寒全論 (The Complete Theory on the *Shang han lun*) which was a copper-type edition differing from the above volumes.

32. *Chien i shang han lun* 簡易傷寒論 (A Simplified *Shang han lun*) by Hokujo Wagasai adopt the style used in the completion of the *Shang han lun chang chu* which consisted of a simplet outline fo the main points from the *Shang han lun.* Other books such as Nakanishi Sinsai's *Shan ting shang han lun* (Revised *shang han lun*); Okubo Jousasu's *Shang han lun ku i* 傷寒論古義 (Early Views on the *Shang han lun*); Ito Osuke's *Shang han lun chang i ting pen* 傷寒論張義定本 (The Exposition of the *Shang han lun*); and Furuya Shihaku's *Fu sheng cheng wen shang han lun* 復聖正文傷寒論 (Restoration of Early Views on the Main Text of the *Shang han lun*) describe only those sections which these authors felt were in the original or main text of the *Shang han lun.*

33. *Chi kuang shang han lun* 輯光傷寒論 (The Compilation and Glorification of the *Shang han lun*) is a copy of

the Upper and Lower Volumes of *Pu cheng chi kuang shang han lun* 補正輯光傷寒論 (A Supplement and Revision to the Compilation and Glorification of the *Shang han lun*). It is the collective effort in Chinese on Yoshimasu Todo's doctrines. Completed by his pupils Fujida Daishin, Tsurada Shin, and Mukida Teki. Even the sentence "Greater yang disease is characterized by a buoyant pulse, stiffness and aching in the head and neck, and chills" was regarded contrary to the views of the early sages and consequently deleted. The end result is greatly simplified volume.

34. *Shang han lun szu chuan* 傷寒論私撰 (A Personal Compilation of the *Shang han lun*), an interpretation by Kohashino Saimenan, is difficult to understand as the author has completely misinterpreted the basic concepts of the *Shang han lun*.

35. *Shang han lun yun yu tu chieh* 傷寒論韵語圖解 (An Illustrative Exposition of the *Shang han lun* in Rhyme) is a unique presentation of the *Shang han lun* by Okada Seian in three volumes.

36. *Shang han lun chu po* 傷寒論舉踣 (Revival of the *Shang han lun*) by Noryo Tienzen is a discussion and explanation of the *Shang han lun* concluded after extensive, specialized research. He was concerned about the etymology of each word and recorded in juxtaposition the changes in the early formulas, folk medicine, and prescriptions of unknown origin.

37. *Shang han lun chien chu* 傷寒論箋註 (The Annotative *Shang han lun*) by Yamahotori Bunhaku is a study of three volumes in Chinese. His research departed from the philosophy of his master Yoshimasu Todo in that it was founded on the *ching-lo* (meridian) concept. The contents of the book is briefly summarized in Chapter Four. Bunhaku points out in the "General Notes": "The three yangs and the three yins were described according to the ancient definition based on the *ching lo* concpet, but it is not absolutely necessary to

restrict the description to one way." He comments further that there was a recent trend to revive Chang Chung-ching's medical theory. Even though Chung-ching's philosophy was closely followed there was no understanding of the value of the formulas. This led eventually to misconceptions about the profound and abstruse meanings of these principles. As a rule, each prescription is intended for a specific purpose. Therefore, if one is not familiar with the overall design of herbal medicine, one can hardly adequately prescribe for the patient's needs.

38. *I chu shang han lun* 翼註傷寒論 (An Annotation of the *Shang han lun*) in Chinese by Miyagihou was completed in five volumes. It is annotated throughout, and includes the main text, notes, and addenda of subsequent research workers.
All of the above books are printed. In addition to these, there are many transcriptions, students' notes and authors' manuscripts, of which a few of the more outstanding follow.

39. *Shang han lun ti sui* 傷寒論剔髓 (Essentials of the *Shang han lun*) by an unknown author is in Chinese and composed of upper and lower volumes. It is helpful to those who are interested in Goto Gonsan's views. It includes annotations from the successors of Gonsan's schools, the phrases often beginning with "Mr. Shoan said" or "Mr. Kouyo said" or "Mr. Kurian said . . . . "

40. *Shang han lun shih* 傷寒論識 (Personal Impressions of the *Shang han lun*) by Asada Sohaku is his research on the *Shang han lun* in Chinese in six volumes divided into seven fascicles. It is extensively annotated with commentaries.
There are also other excellent volumes worth reading such as Mori Tachi's *Shang han lun kao chu* 傷寒論考註 (A Research and Exposition on the *Shang han lun*) and Murai Tsubaki Kotobuki's *Shang han lun chiang lu* 傷寒論講録 (Lectures on *Shang han*

121

lun). These two books are quite long and emphasize verification rather than clinical correlation.

There are also books dealing solely with the herbal prescriptions used in the *Shang han lun* and *Chin kuei yao lueh* which are of value to the researcher. These include Yoshimasu Todo's *Yao cheng* 藥徵 (The Verification of Medicinals); Nakato Hisaken's *Ku fang yao pin kao* 古方藥品考 (Investigation of Ancient Prescription Drugs), and Asada Sohaku's *Ku fang yao i* 古方藥議 (A Discussion on Ancient Prescription Drugs).

Footontes

1.   Sankyo Toyo stated in his *Lun yeh* 論業 (Series of Arguments) that the *Ling shu* and *Su wen* were without a doubt the oldest known medical treatises recorded in *Ching* (Books of History). He had read them from childhood and found them to be of little value in medicine. Toyo felt it ridiculous to study conversations held between Chih Po and Emperor Huang Ti who adulterated the yin-yang theory by disscussing immortality and health hygiene and by misconstruing it with the visceral and *ching-lo* concepts. It was difficult for him to visualize such data being the guide for acupuncture and moxibustion, much less serving as the origin of Chinese medical science.

2.   Todo said in his *I tuan* 醫斷 (Medical Judgments) that the Chinese once regarded the *Nei ching* as being a fabrication compiled in the former Chin period. Different versions of this work appeared after the Six dynasties which should alert the reader to be discriminating. The *Nan ching* is attributed to a Yueh scholar. Its reasonings are unique but, nevertheless, they present great puzzles to medical science. Todo even felt the biography of Pien Ch'iao was spurious.

Chapter Six
The Contents of the *Shang han lun*

The contents of the several earlier editions of the *Shang han lun* vary. This work is based on four of the more well-known, traditional volumes. They are:

a. The Sung edition that was published in the eighth year of Kuanbuan (1668) in Japan. This is comparable to the Sung edition which appeared in China.

b. Cheng's edition, *Annotated Shang han lun*, part of the *Tzu* division of the Imperial Collection of Four Divisions. (The four divisions are *Ching, Shih, Tzu*, and *Chi*.)

c. *Chin kuei yu han ching*, a photocopy of a book that has been in private hands since the early years of the Ching dynasty (1644-1912).

d. Kang ping edition in the author's personal liberary.

Volume by Volume Comparison of the
Four References

The table of contents of the ten volume Sung edition is as follows:

Volume 1. (1) Pulse Diagnosis

123

124

and Treatment of Diseases Following
Perspiration

(18) Identification of Diseases that Cannot
be Treated by the Emetic Method

(19) Identification of Conditions that Can
Be Treated by the Emetic Method

Volume 9. (20) Diagnosis of the Pulses and Confirmations
and Therapy of Diseases that Cannot
Be Treated by the Emetic Method

(21) Diagnosis of the Pulses and Confirmations
of Diseases that Can Be Treated by
the Purgation Method

Volume 10. (22) Identification of the Pulses and Confirmations and Treatment of the Con-
dition Following Perspiration, Emesis,
and Purgation

Cheng Wu-chi's edition also contains ten volumes with a
similar organization to that of the Sung edition. It differs, however, in that the material is rendered into simpler form beginning
with the chapter on "Diagnosis of the Pulses and Confirmations
and Therapy of Diseases That Should Not Be Treated with the
Purgation Method." In the tenth volume modified prescriptions
from the fundamental prescriptions are inserted. Cheng's work
is also annotated and includes a phase movement diagram.

The Ching kuei yu han ching is eight volumes arranged as
follows:

Volume 1.　　　　Comprehensive Notes on Confirmations
and Therapy

Volume 2. (1) Identification of Convulsive, Moisture
and Heatstroke Disorders

(2) Pulse Diagnosis

(3) Identification of the Manifestations, Confirmations, and Treatment of Greater
Yang Disease: Upper Chapter

Volume 3. (4) Identification of the Manifestations, Confirmations, and Treatment of Greater
Yang Disease: Lower Chapter

(5) Identification of the Manifestation, Con-
formations, and Treatment of Sunlight
Yang Disease

125

(6) Identification of the Manifestations, Confirmations, and Treatment of Lesser Yang Disease

Volume 4. (7) Identification of the Manifestations, Confirmations, and Treatment of Greater Yin Disease

(8) Identification of the Manifestations, Confirmations, and Treatment of Lesser Yin Disease

(9) Identification of the Manifestations, Confirmations, and Treatment of Absolute yin Disease

(10) Identification of the Manifestations, Confirmations, and Therapy of Chills, Diarrhea, Vomiting and Hiccoughing

(11) Identification of the Manifestations, Confirmations, and Treatment of Cholera

(12) Identification of the Manifestations, Confirmations, and Treatment of Diseases that Result from Exhaustion Following Recovery from Illness

Volume 5. (13) Identification of the Manifestations, Confirmations, and Treatment of Disease in which the Perspiration Method Is Contraindicated.

(14) Identification of the Manifestations, Confirmations, and Treatment of Conditions in which the Perspiration Method Is Indicated

(15) Identification of the Manifestations, Confirmations, and Treatment of Disease in which the Emetic Method Is Contraindicated

(16) Identification of the Manifestations, Confirmations, and Treatment of Conditions in which the Emetic Method Is Indicated

(17) Identification of the Manifestations, Confirmations, and Treatment of Diseases in which the Purgation Method Is Contraindicated

ditions Stemming from Recovery, and
Fatal Diseases

Volume 7. Methods Used in Processing and Preparing Herbs

Volume 8. Methods Used in Processing and Preparing Herbs (continued)

The Kang Ping edition is more ambiguous in its content
as is evident from its table of contents.

Notes on the *Shang han lun*

Identification of Greater Yang Disease and Convulsive,
Moisture, and Heatstroke Conditions

Identification of Greater Yang Disease

Identification of Greater Yang Disease — Chest Binding
Conditions

Identification of Sunlight Yang Disease

Identification of Lesser Yang Disease

Identification of Greater Yin Disease

Identification of Lesser Yin Disease

Identification of Absolute Yin Disease

Identification of Absolute Yin Conditions: Cholera

Identification of Diseases due to Fatigue after Recovery
from an Illness

From the table of contents of these four basic references,
it is evident that both the chapters on "Identification of the
Pulses" and "Pulses in the Healthy Individual" were recorded in
Sung and Ching editions. Only the chapter on "Identification
of the Pulses" was included in the second volume of *Chin kuei
yu han ching* while neither chapter appeared in the Kang Ping
edition. These two chapters belong to a completely different
system from that of the main theory of the *Shang han lun*, a
fact that has been well documented in detail in the section "Exploration of the *Shang han lun* in the Kang Ping edition."[1] Taki
Genkan felt that they were added to the *Shang han lun* by Wang
Shu-ho who had summarized them from various sources.
Tachibana Haruki was also of the opinion that these two chapters
differed from the concepts on the definition of pulses expressed
in the *Shang han lun* but felt they were similar to those described
by Wang Shu-ho in his "Classic on the Pulses". This leads to the
conclusion that these chapters were added by subsequent investigators who referred to Wang's work, or that Wang himself

used these chapters to help complete the classic. However.
Kawaetsu Koozan feels that these chapters were appended by
Kao Chi-cheng when he was revising the *Shang han lun*. Otsuka
also suggests that Kao might have discovered Chang Chung-
ching's "Pulse Theory" and added it to the *Shang han lun*. This
is emphasized in the section on the *Shang han lun* and Chang
Chung-ching found in the present work.

Wang Su-ho's "Notes on the *Shang han*" outlines a different
system from that in the *Shang han lun*, yet it is found in the
beginning of the second volume of the Sung and Cheng editions,
and at the commencement of the table of contents in the Kang
Ping version. The "Notes on the *Shang han*" have been replaced
by "General Notes on Confirmations and Treatment" in the first
volume of the *Yu han ching*. The notes are comparable to the
context and style of *Chien chin yao feng* (Thousand Golden
Prescriptions) of the T'ang dynasty, another reason for suggesting
that this portion could have been added by a researcher in the
Sui-T'ang Periods.

The Sung and Cheng editions and *Yu han ching* all contain
the chapter on "Identification of the Pulses and Confirmations of
Convulsive, Moisture and Heatstroke Diseases". A similar chapter
entitled "Identification of *Tai yang ping* (Greater Yang Disease):
Convulsions, Moisture and Heatstroke" is also included in the
Kang Ping edition. The Sung version, however, substitutes the
word "malaria" for convulsions. This same section is well covered
by the same title in the *Chin kuei yao lueh* (Prescriptions within
the Golden Chamber) which raises the question of why it was
included in the *Shang han lun*. Otsuka suggests that this is because the symptoms of *tai yang ping* (greater yang disease) are
included in all editions but the Kang Ping where it appears as
"*tai yang ping*." The symptoms are very similar to those of
"Convulsions, Moisture and Heatstroke." It should more appropriately be recorded as "Identification of the Convulsive, Moisture and Heatstroke Diseases of the Greater Yang Conditions."

Here the word "*ching*" (convulsion) refers to such conditions as tetanus, etc., which are often associated with seizures;
"*shih*" (moisture) signifies diseases such as rheumatism, neuralgia,
etc.; and "*yeh*" (heatstroke) indicates illnesses due to overexpo-
sure to the sun.

The eight chapters after the one on "Identification of the

Pulses and Confirmations and Treatment of Diseases in which Perspiration Method Is Contraindicated" were added after the seventh volume in the Sung and Cheng editions. The ten chapters from the "Identification of the Pulses, Confirmation and Therapy of the Warm Diseases" were included after the sixth volume in the *Yu han ching.*

*The chapter*s on "The Processing Methods for Herbs and Prescriptions": are included in the seventh and eighth volumes of the *Yu han ching.* Among these prescriptions there are a few not included in the other editions, such as *Tiao-chi-yin, Chu-tu-huang-lien-wan* (Pig Stomach and Coptis Formula), and *Ching-mu-hsiang-wan* (Birthwort and Pharbitis Formula) which may have been first used in the Sui and T'ang dynasties.

Discussion of the Chapters on the Three Yins and the Three Yangs

The main text of the *Shang han lun* begins with the chapter on the "Identification of the Greater Yang Diseases" and concludes with a review of absolute yin disease. We find that the initial chapters on greater yang disease occupy half of the entire contents. This does not signify its greater importance, rather greater yang disease is analyzed from the standpoint of diagnosis, treatment and the derivation of various yang and yin diseases from the greater yang condition. Also the greater yang diseases are described in three chapters, viz. the upper, middle and lower chapters under the same title.

The greater yang disease section is followed successively by chapters on sunlight yang and lesser yang diseases. Although the latter is quite short, it does not lessen its importance. It is only because much information on this condition already appears with the greater yang disease material, thus obviating its repetition. The same holds true with the chapter on the absolute yin disease, the data having been fully reviewed in the greater and absolute yin disease chapters.

A review of the chapters on the yin and yang disease will show that they are not independent but interrelated. In his "Ancestral Doctrines of Medical Science", Wutsuki Kondai stressed that the *Shang han lun* should be read as a unit. A con-

130

trary point of view was expressed by Tod Yoshimasu who pointed out in *Chi kuang shang han lun* 輯光傷寒論 (The Compilation and Glorification of the *Shang han lun*) that the various chapters are independent and can be read and understood without referring to each other. Otsuka supports Kondai's viewpoint because the contents are so interwoven to demonstrate the extreme, complex variation in the diseases, therefore one must read the entire text to correlate the various aspects presented.

The *Shang han lun* adopted the classification of the yin and yang disease from the six meridian conditions of the *Su wen* but with a slightly different connotation. In this respect, Yamada Seishin states in "A Research on the *Shang han lun*" that Chang Chung-ching used the three yin and the three yang system to explain the external and internal confirmations and the corresponding pulses; he also used the febrile disease theory found in the *Su wen* but with a different twist. Otsuka studied this situation and found that aching pain in the head and neck and rigidity of the spine and limbs are the characteristic symptoms found during the first day of greater yang disease and conform to the indications and confirmation of Chang Chung-ching's *Ma-huang-tang* (*Ma-huang* Combination). Somatic fever, aching in the eyes, dryness of the nose, and inability to lie down typify the second day manifestations of sunlight yang disease, representing the indications and confirmation of Chang Chung-ching's *Ta-ching-lung-tang* (Major Blue Dragon Combination). Both are external confirmations. The thoraco-costal discomfort and deafness present on the third day of lesser yang disease is Chang's *Hsiao-chai-hu-tang* (Minor Bupleurum Combination) confirmation, which signifies the semi-external confirmation. Symptoms contracted the fourth day of greater yin or the other yin diseases include abdominal distention; dryness of the throat, mouth, or tongue; irritability and stuffiness; and contraction of the scrotum. They correspond to *Ta-cheng-chi-tang* (Rhubarb Combination) confirmation and represent the internal confirmation regardless of whether the symptoms are mild or severe. The rules of treatment call for perspiration for the three yang diseases and purgation for the three yin conditions, there being no other therapy. Although these two methods are different, they are both used to treat diseases of "firm fever." Chang Chung-ching, therefore, made an approximate grouping by including such dis-

131

eases in the chapters on the three yangs. However, illnesses due to mild chills were included in the section on three yins. This made it easy to discriminate between yin and yang, for without doing so, the diseases associated with mild chills could not otherwise be classified.

Yakazu Arimichi also states in his *Han fang i hsueh tsung lun* 漢方醫學總論 (A General Exposition on Chinese Medicine) that the locations of the three yins and three yangs as found in the *Shang han lun* are in agreement with the three yin and the three yang meridians, e.g. greater yang diseases occur at such locations where the greater yang (foot) and urinary bladder and greater yang (hand) and small intestine meridians pass through their respective pathways. Also, lesser yang conditions result where the lesser yang (foot) and gall bladder and lesser yang (hand) and *san chiao* meridians circulate. Sunlight yang illnesses are evident at areas corresponding to the pathways of the sunlight (foot) and stomach and sunlight yang (hand) and colon meridians. Similarly, greater yin disease occurs in locations associated with the channels of the greater yin (foot) and spleen and greater yin (hand) and lung meridians; lesser yin illnesses involve the lesser yin (foot) and kidney and lesser yin (hand) and heart circuits; and absolute yin conditions implicate the absolute (foot) and liver and absolute yin (hand) and pericardium pathways. The manifestations of diseases are more evident at the three foot-yin and three foot-yang meridians than at the three hand-yin and three hand-yang circuits.

If the three yang and the three yin diseases are regarded as the warp, then *chung feng* (colds) and *shang han* (febrile diseases) represent the woof, crossing and interweaving with the warp. *Chung feng* is associated with mild or benign illnesses, whereas *shang han* indicates more severe or malignant conditions. *Shang han* cases may progress rapidly and if treatment is delayed result in serious and grave symptoms. The febrile conditions (*shang han*) described in conjunction with the three yangs and the three yins are comparable to those discussed in Chapter Three of Otsuka's work but differ from those mentioned in the "Notes" appended to the *Shang han* chapter by Wang Su-ho.

As previously noted, the *Shang han lun* covers changes in various diseases; their genesis, development, and completion; methodology; rules; and therapy in a manner quite unknown in previous or subsequent works. It is also well to emphasize the merit of the many references and annotations added by Wang Shu-ho and succeeding researchers in the several chapters on the three yangs and the three yins.

Distinction of the Original Text from the Supplementary Expositions and Annotations

When reading the *Shang han lun*, one occasionally encounters the phrase "It is doubtful if" which is followed by additional statements such as "This is Chung-ching's prescription" or "This is Chung-ching's way" or "It is Chung-ching who. . ." These words were regarded as additions of unknown authors to the Kang Ping editions. However, if we assume them to have been added before the Sung dynasty, then we can be certain that these later versions differ from the original. Otsuka discussed the various aspects of this situation in Chapter Three and further commented that the problem concerning subsequent alteration of the *Shang han lun* had existed from ancient times. Moreover, whenever the interpretation of a passage in the *Shang han lun* appeared to be paradoxical or difficult to comprehend, it was often felt to be redundant or incorrectly placed in the text and consequently deleted. Also Fang Yu-chih of the Ming dynasty, author of *Shang han lun tiao pien* 傷寒論條辯 (Monographical Identification of the *Shang han lun*), stated that the actual form of the original work was completely altered by Wang Su-ho and for this reason he was regarded by some as a betrayer of Chang Chung-ching.

In the Preface of the *Revised Edition of the Monographical Identification of the Shang han lun* 重刻傷寒論條辨序 , one reads that in the past there were numerous annotations on Chang Chung-ching's writings such as Wang Shu-ho of the Chin 晉 dynasty, Cheng Wu-chi of the Chin 金 dynasty, Kao Pao-heng and Lin I of the Sung dynasty, et al. Wang's version resulted in a complete revision and clarified alteration of the basic text with insertion of his own viewpoint as desired.

As previously mentioned, Sorai has led the movement to resore the original *Shang han lun* to its proper place in medical history. This was well illustrated in *The Orthodox Shang han lun* 正文傷寒論 , *The Original Shang han lun* 原文傷寒論 , and other publications in which he criticizes other altered editions that appeared in and after Wang Shu-ho's time.

Hakumizu Tannayoshi, who authored *Liu's Shang han lun* 傷寒論劉氏傳 divided the *Shang han lun* into the main text, Chang Chung-ching's comments, and the annotations of subsequent writers. The main text consisted of sixty-six monographs on methods of treatment collected from early times and attributed to Pien Ch'iao, Ch'un-yu I, et al. Chang Chung-ching's section contained two hundred and two essays on illustrative cases of these various available methods of therapy. The total two hundred sixty-eight—all written by Chang Chung-ching—were regarded as the original work. The annotations consisted of one hundred eighteen articles contributed by investigators after the Chin and T'ang dynasties.

Saiseisai's students compiled *A Specific Interpretation of the Shang han lun* 傷寒論特解 which comprises three hundred ninety monographs, one hundred twenty of which embrace the main text with appendices containing the remainder. It was felt that the original text was simple, concise, forceful, and expressive as opposed to the other text which appeared fragmented, redundant, ponderous, and stilted. However, this is probably true as subsequent researchers often adulterated the original text with annotations and comments, which if deleted restores the pristine nature of the primary work.

Nakanishi Seisai in his "Identification and Verification of the *Shang han lun*" 傷寒論辯正 also points out some portions of the main editions came from later investigators. This opinion was shared by Asada Sohaku who in his "My Opinions about the *Shang han lun*" 傷寒論識 discusses various portions of the text which had been altered.

Further, the explanation of the terms yin and yang as used in the primary and subsequent editions have come to have different connotations.

Footnotes

1. The two chapters "Pulse Identification" and "Pulses in a Healthy Individual" as recorded in "An Extra-Historical

Record of the *Shang han lun*" 傷寒論外傳 suggest a pulse theory which differs from the main text. The style consists of four to six word rhymes that vary from the ancient text and suggest the more flamboyant structure of subsequent writers whose work as similar to that of Wang Shu-ho's. It may well be that subsequent researchers wrote these two chapters, or conversely, Wang way have compiled his pulse theory on this information. However, as their interpretations differ from the main text, they should be separated.

2. Kawaetsu Kosan, *Shang han lun mo cheng shih* 傷寒論脈證式 (The Pulses and Confirmation of the *Shang han lun*).

3. *Journal of the Japanese Oriental Medical Society* 日本東洋醫學會誌 Vol. 5 No. 1.

4. *Exploration of the Shang han lun of the Kang Ping Edition:* 康平傷寒論之發掘 Chapter 4, Section 4.

Chapter Seven
Herbs Used in the *Shang han lun*

Efficacy and Processing of Medicinals

The medicinals recorded in the *Shang han lun* number slightly over ninety, far fewer than those included in the *Chin kuei yao lueh*. The efficacy and processing of these medicinals will be discussed briefly in this section.[1]

Cheng Pan-hsien's concise and concrete descriptions of the herbs as found in *Hsin pen ts'ao pei yao* 新本草備要 (hereafter referred to as the *Pei yao*) will be quoted relative to their usefulness.

Aconite 附子

This herb is the young root of *Aconitum carmichaeli* Debx. of the Ranunculaceae family. (The mother root is *wu tou;* the young annexed rootlet, *fu tzu;* the rootlet that grows alongside of *fu tzu, cheh tzu;* the long slender rootlet, *tien hsiung;* and the forked rootlet, *wu huei.* These five parts come from the same plant but are named differently.) It is a poisonous plant, and if dosage is inaccurate, poisoning invariably results, sometimes even fatal poisoning. When appropriately used, however, it has an outstanding effect and is one of the truly essential drugs of Chinese medicine.

The *Pei yao* records, "It is used as a cardiac tonic and a stimulant, diuretic and diaphoretic, and for chronic dyspepsia." It also has analgesic, anticonvulsant, cardiotonic, and spermatonic actions and is indispensable for patients with a yin confirmation.

Aconite is used in either the raw or fired state. In both methods, "Aconite is peeled and divided into eight pieces." In the "fired" processing method, the aconite is wrapped in thick moistened paper and embedded in a heap of ashes under a hot fire, thereby enabling the poisonous constituent, aconitine alkaloid, to undergo chemical decomposition.

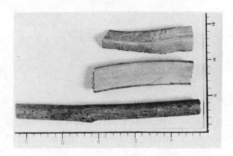

Akebia 通草（木通）

Also known as *mu tung,* this drug is derived from the stem of *Akebia quinata* Decne. of the Lardizabalaceae family. It has diuretic effect.

Alisma 澤瀉

This drug is the tuber of *Alisma plantago — aquatica* L. of the Alismataceae family. (The Chinese name is derived from its ability to discharge water.) It is recorded in the *Pei yao* that it is used for edema, dysuria, and heatstroke. In addition to its diuretic effect, this drug is also effective in quenching thirst and relieving giddiness. The latter term connotes the dizzy feeling of being compressed by something.

Allium (White Stem of Ciboule) 葱白

This is the white stem of *Allium fistulosum* L. of the Liliaceae family. The *Pei yao* records that it is "used as an expectorant and stimulant and as a diaphoretic, diuretic, hemostatic, and anthelmintic agent; externally it is applied on abscesses, ulcers, and gout."

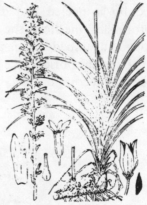

Anemarrhena 知母

This drug is the rhizome of *Anemarrhena asphodeloides* Bge. of the Liliaceae family. The *Pei yao* indicates that it is "used as an antipyretic, a sedative, and a diuretic."

Anemone 白頭翁

This drug is the root of *Anemone cernua* Thunb. of the Ranunculaceae family. (The hair-like filaments hanging down from the apices of the violet stamens behind the flower resemble an old man's hair, and its Chinese name is derived from this characteristic.) The *Pei yao* lists its functions as being "used to cleanse the heat and cool the blood in amenorrhea and febrile diarrhea." In other words, this drug has analgesic, anti-inflammatory, astringent, and hemostatic effects.

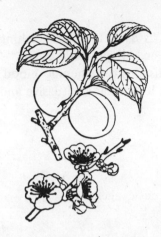

Apricot Seed 杏仁

This drug is derived from the kernel of the seed of *Prunus armeniaca* L. of the Rosaceae family. The *Pei yao* records, "It is used as an antitussive, expectorant, and flavoring agent." It is also helpful in treating stagnancy of blood, as a diuretic in reducing edema, and as an analgesic. It has an aridity-moisture effect.

The processing methods utilized for apricot seeds are either "soaking in water to remove the outer skin, apex, and the twin kernels" or "removing the skin and apex and cooking till they are dry." However, modern practice consists of removing the skins and apices only and then chopping the kernels into pieces.

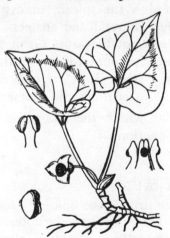

Asarum 細辛

This drug is the root of *Asarum sieboldi* Miq. of the Aristolochiaceae family. Another species called *tu hsi hsin* (*Asarum blumei* Duch.) is not the genuine variety. The *Pei yao* indicates that it "is used for facial aching due to colds; it is also an anti-pyretic and diaphoretic agent." Asarum is effective in adjusting metabolism, strengthening blood circulation, and increasing urine volume. It also has antitussive and analgesic actions.

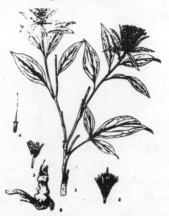

Atractylodes 白朮

This herb is the rhizome of *Atractylodes ovata* Thunb. of the Compositae family. In Japan the old roots of atractylodes are called *tsang chu*, and the big, fleshy, young, tender rhizomes are designated *pai chu*.

The functions of atractylodes, as noted in the *Pei yao*, are "to replenish the spleen, to dry up dampness, and to use as a stomachic, diuretic and analgesic agent." The spleen in Chinese medicine is not the same organ as in modern Western medicine. They use the word to denote the digestive function of the alimentary system. Thus atractylodes works to promote digestive action, to strengthen the stomach, to dispel pathological water stagnating within the body, and to reduce fever. It also has an analgesic action.

Bakeri 薤白

This drug is the bulb of *Allium bakeri* Regel of the Liliaceae family. The *Ming i pei lu* notes, "Baker's garlic is bitter in taste and warm natured. It acts to eliminate cold and heat, to exclude moisture, to warm the interior, and to disperse coagulation." Here "interior" refers to the internal portions of the body. This drug is capable of dispersing coagulations, treating thoracic and back-aches, and promoting diuresis.

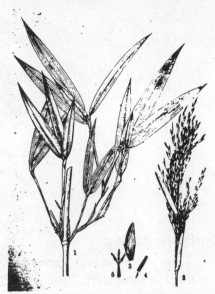

Bamboo Leaves 竹葉

This drug is derived from the leaves of *Pleioblastus amarus* Keng F. of the Gramineae family. It has sedative, anti-tussive, diuretic, and analgesic effects and can also alleviate "ascending *chi*."

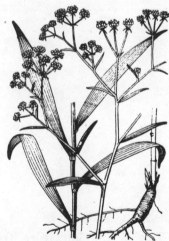

Bupleurum 柴胡

This drug is the root of *Bupleurum falcatum* L. of the Umbelliferae family. *The Pei yao* records that it "is an antipyretic and is especially effective against malaria," which is not correct. Bupleurum can fortify the functions of the liver and treat thoracocostal distress. It has antipyretic, analgesic, tranquilizing, and diuretic effects. It is merely cut into slices for use and entails no special processing.

141

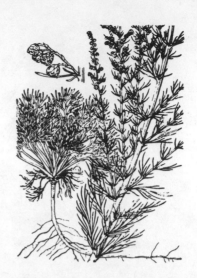

Capillaris 茵陳蒿

This is the young leaves of *Artemisia capillaris* Th. of the Compositae family. In Japan, the fruit only is used. The *Pei yao* records, "It treats rheumatism, renders diuresis, and is an important remedy for jaundice." This drug has antiphlogistic, diuretic, and cholegogueous effects and is beneficial in hepatic disorders.

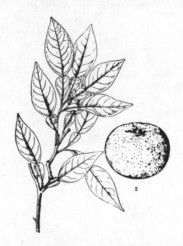

Chih-Shih 枳實

This is the immature fruit of *Poncirus trifoliata* Raf. of the Rutaceae family which grows in China. In Japan they use the immature fruit of *Citrus aurantium* L. The *Pei yao* says, "It has expectorant, diaphoretic, diuretic, and digestive effects." It is an aromatic, stomachic agent with a relaxing action on muscle tension.

The processing method for this drug comprises "immersion in water and baking until yellow." Water immersion is necessary to

142

render the fruit soft, otherwise it remains very hard; the baking until yellow results in drying the drug.

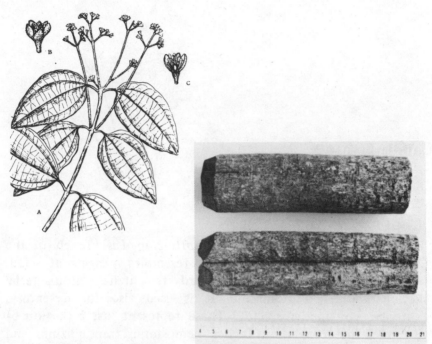

Cinnamon 桂枝、桂皮

This herb comes from the bark of the branches or twigs of *Cinnamomum cassia* Bl. of the Lauraceae family, which grows in Southern China, Southeast Asia, and Eastern India. It is not derived from the bark of the trunk but only from that of the smaller branches. Inaba Wagamizo said, "Cinnamon is the bark from the small twigs, not from the coarse trunks." It is stated in the *Pei yao* that it "acts to render diaphoresis, to harmonize the blood vessels and skin capillaries, and to treat an adverse up-rush." It is an important drug for these symptoms. Cinnamon causes sweating which dispels surface toxins; circulates blood and *ch'i*; harmonizes yin and yang; and treats up–rushing of *ch'i*.

It is processed by removing the skin. This sounds paradoxical. Since the skin is the bark which is used for medicine, how can it be removed? Actually, it is only the tasteless, odorless, superficial, coarse layer that must be removed.

143

Clear Wine 清酒

Wine is used as a stimulant to enhance blood circulation and to promote the absorption of medicines.

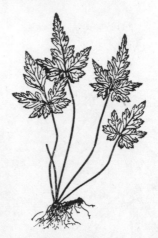

Coptis 黃連

This drug is the root of *Coptis chinensis* Franch. of the Ranunculaceae family. (The root resembles a string of small, yellowish balls.) The *Pei yao* records that it has "antibacterial action and is a stomachic. It is used also for dysentery, enteritis, conjunctivitis, etc." These represent just a portion of its medicinal properties. It has hemostatic, tranquilizing, and antiphlogistic effects and is applicable for "flush-up," excitement, hemorrhage, and inflammation.

The commercial form comes in slices, the hair-like roots having been burned away.

Croton 巴豆

Croton is the seed of *Croton tiglium* L. of the Euphoribiaceae family. The *Pei yao* says this drug is processed by "removing the skin and core, cooking until it becomes dark, then grinding to a paste or ointment." In other words, the epithelium and germ are first removed; the seeds are then cooked with boiled glutinous rice until the mixture darkens; and finally the meal is placed in a mortar and ground into a putty-like ointment.

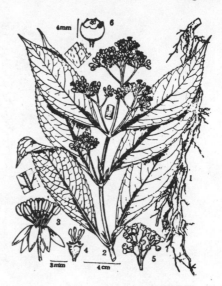

Dichroa 蜀漆

This is the leaves and stalks of young shoots of *Dichroa febrifuga* Lour. of the Saxifragaceae family. The *Pei yao* mentions that it is used "to intercept malaria" meaning to cut out the fever associated with the condition. The drug also has a sedative effect.

It is processed by washing until it is free from its fishy odor.

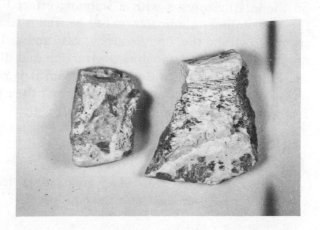

Dragon Bone 龍骨

This is the fossilized bones of ancient mammals. The *Pei yao* states that it is used as a tranquilizer, hypnotic, and tonic. That is, it can relieve the palpitation consequent to nervousness and hypersensitivity, and alleviate anxiety.

145

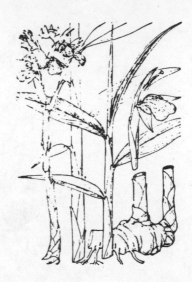

Dry Ginger 乾薑

This is the dried root of *Zingiber officinale* Rosc. of the Zingiberaceae family. In the *Pei yao* it indicates that it "warms the insides and removes chills, dries dampness, eliminates sputum, and aids digestion by relieving flatulence." Here the word "insides" refers to the internal part of the body or viscera; sputum denotes pathological water or fluid. Thus ginger has a stimulating action on the internal organs with a warming effect besides. It adjusts the metabolism, eliminates excessive fluids that have become stagnant within the body, dispels gas, and aids digestion. The drug is helpful in eliminating obstruction and distention beneath the heart; thus it has a stomachic action. It is prepared commercially by removing the soft cork layer and then used in slices. No further processing is necessary.

Egg Yolk 雞子黃

The *Pei yao* records, "Egg yolk cleans heat, nourishes the yin, and is used as an analgesic and antidote."

Euphorbia 大戟

Euphorbia is the root of *Euphorbia pekinensis* Rupr. of the Euphorbiaceae family. It is a diuretic and a cathartic. The *Pei yao* says, "It is used primarily for cathartic action but also for water stagnation." Here the latter term means water toxin (edema).

Evodia 吳茱萸

This drug is the fruit of *Evodia rutaecarpa* (Juss.) Bth. of the Rutaceae family. The *Pei yao* records that it "acts to remove the toxins of wind, cold and moisture, to descend *ch'i*, and to relieve depression and occlusion. It is used as a stimulant, carminative, astringent, and anthelmintic." Wind and cold are external toxins, while moisture is an internal toxin. Thus this drug treats the up-rushing of *ch'i*, removes the stagnation and occlusion of *ch'i*, functions as a stimulant to agitate sedimented stagnation, removes gases within the intestine, astringes and kills parasites. It is effective as a stomachic, analgesic, and diuretic and is helpful for headaches and vomiting.

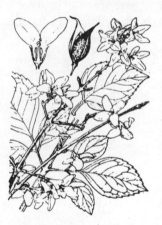

Forsythia 連翹

This is the root of *Forsythia suspensa* Vahl. of the Oleaceae family. Its fruit is called *lien chiao*. In the *Pei yao* it says, "It is used internally for scabies and other ulcers." In the *Shang han lun*, forsythia is noted to be the root of *lien chiao*. It has diuretic and anti-inflammatory actions and is good for skin diseases.

Fraxinus 秦皮

This is the bark of the *Fraxinus bungeana* DC. of the Olea-ceae family. The *Pei yao* states. "It is used as a remedy for eye diseases." Its action is anti-inflammatory, antipyretic, astringent.

147

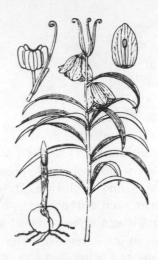

Fritillaria 貝母

This is the scaly bulb of *Fritillaria roylei* Hook. of the Liliaceae family. (The Chinese name is derived from the fleshy bulbs that resemble a number of cowry shells.) The *Pei yao* says, "It is used specifically as an expectorant and analgesic." It resembles platycodon in its therapeutic action.

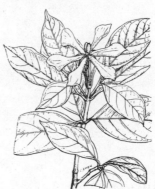

Gardenia 栀子

This drug is also known as *shan chih tzu* and is the fruit of *Gardenia jasminoides* Ellis, *Gardenia florida* L. of the Rubiaceae family. The *Pei yao* notes that it "corrects blood disorders, purges fire, and stops bleeding and severe vomiting." Thus gardenia treats somatic fever, thoracic distress and stuffiness, heart and chest pains and has tranquilizing, hemostatic, antiphlogistic, diuretic, antipyretic, and mild laxative effects.

It is processed by wedging open or breaking up the fruit.

Gelatin 阿膠

This glue-like substance comes from the hides of cows and donkeys. (The best quality gelatin is made by cooking the hides in the water from a well located 60 miles northeast of Yang Ker Prefecture in Shangtung Province, which was called the Ah Prefecture in former times.) The *Pei yao* records that it is a "nourishing, enriching, moistening, and supplementing agent. It is also a hemostatic for the treatment of external wounds such as bruises, injuries, and burns." In summary, this drug has nourishing, enriching, strengthening, hemostatic, alleviating, and tranquilizing effects.

Genkwa 芫花

This drug is the flower bud of *Daphne genkwa* S. et Z. of the Thymelaeaceae family. The *Pei yao* states that it is "used for edema and removal of sputum." It is used after being cooked.

Ginger 生薑

Ginger is the rhizome of *Zingiber officinale* Rosc. of the Zingiberaceae family. It is not peeled but used as presented. The *Pei yao* states that it is "used as a stomachic and antiemetic. The skin of ginger moves water (diuretic); hence it is prescribed for dropsy and tumidity (swellings)." It is an aromatic stomachic and antiemetic which strengthens water metabolism within the body and helps reduce swellings and abdominal fullness.

The ginger employed in cooking is the fresh rhizome, while that used in medicine is of the dry variety.

Ginseng 人參

Ginseng is the root of *Panax ginseng* C. A. Meyer of the Araliaceae family. It is so named because its form resembles that of the human body. The uses of this herb as recorded in the *Pei yao* are as "a tonic for pulmonary phthisis, neurasthenia, impotence, spermatorrhea, senility, anemia, nephrosis, metropathy, and all other debilitating diseases that exhaust the body strength. It is especially efficacious for neurasthenic headaches and vertigo. It stimulates the metabolism of the body, especially

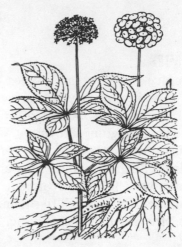

that related to carbohydrates. It also has a diuretic effect." In addition, it improves digestion and promotes absorption by increasing the appetite and reducing vomiting and diarrhea.

Gypsum 石膏

This drug, also called *han sui shih* (cold water stone), is naturally occurring calcium sulfate hydrate. The *Pei yao* records its functions as follows: "It is used as a cleaning and cooling agent for fevers. It is also helpful in tranquilizing and in suppressing thirst."

The processing method for gypsum is recorded as "crushing and wrapping it in a linen." In the time of the writing of the *Shang han lun* linen was not woven from cotton or mulberry but was made from silk. Hence silk linen is used to wrap the crushed gypsum for decoction.

Haematite 代赭石

This is a naturally occurring red iron ore found in the Tai prefecture of Shansi province for which this drug is named in Chinese. According to the *Pei yao,* it is used as an astringent. In addition, it has hematopoietic and hemostatic properties.

Hirudo (Leech) 水蛭

Also known as *ma huang* (螞蟥), this drug is found in fresh water, usually rivers. It has the ability to dissolve old blood clots.

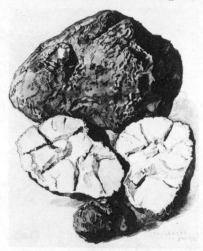

Hoelen 茯苓

This drug is derived from the underground fungi of the Polyporus family, a parasite found on the roots of pine trees which forms into a big lump or massive ball. (It was originally named *fu ling* which literally meant "hidden spirit." It was believed in ancient times the holy spirit of the pine hid on the roots and formed a large mass.) The functions, as recorded in the *Pei yao,* state that it "is used as a diuretic to treat edema and urinary stuttering. It is also a tonic for the debilitated. The skin of hoelen is specifically capable of moving water, hence is indicated for dropsy and skin edema." The term "urinary stuttering" is used here to imply general diseases which involve the bladder, prostate gland, and urethra. It does not denote gonorrhea as it would in modern medicine. Skin edema refers to the swelling found in dropsy. This drug also has a calming effect for excitement and palpitation. It is used in slices without further processing.

Inula 旋覆花

This drug is the flower of *Inula britannica* DC. of the Compositae family. (The flowers are green and grow lushly and luxuriantly in the form of a large, round cover.) It is recorded in the *Pei yao* that it "is used to descend *ch'i* and remove sputum, and also as a stomachic and expectorant." The word sputum as used here denotes "water toxin."

151

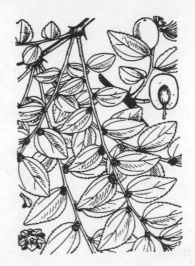

Jujube 大棗

Jujube is the fruit of *Zizyphus vulgaris* Lam. of the Rhamnaceae family. Its efficacies are recorded in the *Pei yao* as follows: "It is used as a paregoric and as a tonic." Thus it has the same action as licorice in mollifying the various drugs. In addition, it has a strengthening effect and is used for severe coughs, abdominal discomfort, cramps, and cardiac palpitation.

The recorded processing method for jujube is "wedging." Each fruit is wedged open with a small knife. However, this way has been replaced by a cutting procedure since it was too time consuming to be practical.

Kan-sui 甘遂

This herb is the rhizome of *Euphorbia kansui* Liou of the Euphorbiaceae family. In the *Pei yao* it is reported useful for "treating dropsy." It is a cathartic and also has diuretic properties.

Kaolin 赤石脂

This drug is the red variety of siliceous clay that contains iron oxide. It has antidiarrheal and hemostatic effects. The *Pei yao* mentions that it is used as an astringent. It is pulverized before use.

Lepidium 葶藶子

This is the fruit of *Lepidium apetalum* Willd of the Cruciferae family. The *Pei yao* mentions that it is used as a diuretic and expectorant. It is used only after it has been cooked.

Licorice 甘草

Licorice is the root of *Glycyrrhiza glabra* L. of the Leguminosae family. It harmonizes all drugs and detoxifies the adverse effects of herbs; hence it is also designated "the country's elder." The *Pei yao* records, "It is used as a flavoring agent to mollify various drugs, and to treat coughs and sore throat. It works synergistically with other drugs." In other words, it is recommended for the alleviation of acute and intermittent aching, convulsions, and coughs; it also is a flavoring agent for bitter herbs and acts synergistically with other drugs. It further has a hepatonic and detoxifying action. For use, the crude drug is merely sliced or else baked and then cut into pieces.

Limonite (*Tai-i-yu-yu-liang*) 太一禹餘糧

This drug's name is derived from the legend that says it is a fossil of the food left behind by the troops of Yu after a triumphant battle. It is a putty iron ore. The *Pei yao* says, "It is used specifically for hemostasis, anemia, and emaciating jaundice." It has astringent, hemostatic, and antidiarrheal effects. It is crushed or ground into fine pieces before use.

Linum 麻仁

This drug is also called *ma tzu jen* and is the seed of *Cannabis sativa* L. of the Moraceae family. It is an emollient laxative. Presently, this herb has been substituted by *Linum usitatissimum* L.

Magnolia Bark 厚朴

This is the bark from the branches of *Magnolia officinalis* Reh. & Wil. of the Magnoliaceae family. The *Pei yao* states that it "is also a stomachic and diuretic." The drug thus treats up-

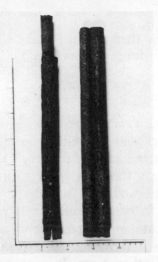
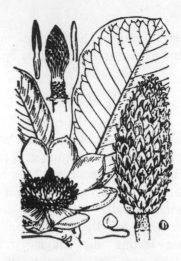

rushing *ch'i,* making it fluent and relaxed, and also relieves the muscle tension that accompanies convulsions. In a manner similar to that used for licorice and cinnamon, it is processed by baking which enables the outer cork layer to be removed.

Ma-huang 麻黃

This is the part of *Ephedra sinica* Stapf. of the Ephedraceae family that grows above ground. The *Pei yao* records, "It is a sympathetic stimulant used exclusively for diaphoresis and the removal of bronchial spasm in asthma. The root of *ma-huang* is antihidrotic." From this we learn that *ma-huang* has a sympathomimetic action, promotes sweating, and treats stridor. It also acts as a diuretic and is useful in the treatment of muscular and articular pain.

It is processed by removing the nodes from the stems which appear above the ground. It is said that these nodes are antihidrotic. Commercially the product is sold in short lengths, cut from the stems, with the nodes attached.

Maltose 膠飴

This is the maltose syrup or jelly produced by cooking rice and wheat germ together. It is also called *I tang.* In the *Pei yao* it says, "It is used to supplement debility and benefit vitality." Thus this drug has nourishing and strengthening effects and also acts as a paregoric.

Mel (also called "white honey") 食蜜

This is ordinary bee's honey, also known as white honey. It has nourishing, strengthening, and paregoric effects.

Melon Pedicle 瓜蒂

This drug is the peduncle of *Cucumis melo* L. of the Cucurbitaceae family. However, since the peduncles from the varieties of melons now cultivated do not have a very bitter taste, they cannot be used as an emetic. The melon pedicle gathered in ancient times belonged to another variety of sweet melon not found today. It is processed by cooking to a yellow color.

Minium 鉛丹

This is red lead oxide. It is included in the prescription *Chai-hu-chia-lung-ku-mu-li-tang*. Keisetsu used it in one case which resulted in lead poisoning with protracted drooling. Accordingly, he, Asada Dohaku et al. have discontinued its use.

Mirabilitum 芒硝

Generally, sodium sulfate is used in place of mirabilitum. However, pharmacognostical research carried out at the Seisoryin Institute has established that the mirabilitum used in ancient times was actually magnesium sulfate. It has diuretic and cathartic actions.

Mume 烏梅

This is the immature fruit of *Prunus mume* S. et Z. of the Rosaceae family. It is smoked with bituminous coal. It treats vomiting, descends *ch'i*, removes heat, and tranquilizes, besides being anthelmintic (ascariasis).

Ophiopogon 麥門冬

This drug is the swollen, tuber-like portion of the root of *Ophiopogon japonicus* Ker.-Gawl of the Liliaceae family. It is noted in *Pei yao* that it "is used as a nourisher, a paregoric, an

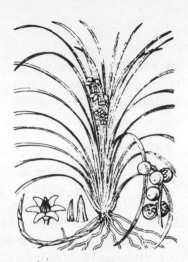

expectorant, and as an antipyretic agent." In addition, it also has enriching, moistening, and diuretic effects.

It is processed by "removing the heart": the hard, thread-like central core of the root. However, since the war the decored form is no longer available.

Oryza 粳米

This is the unhulled rice of *Oryza sativa* L. of the Gramineae family. It has nourishing, paregoric, and thirst-quenching effects.

Oyster Shell 牡蠣

This drug is the shells of *Ostrea* of the Ostreidae family. (All genera of clams or shell fish are either oviparous or viviparous, except this species which is born through metamorphosis and is exclusively of the male gender.) The *Pei yao* states, "It is used as an antacid stomachic." It is effective in tranquilizing and strengthening. It is processed by roasting and baking.

Paeonia 芍藥

Peony is the root of *Paeonia albiflora* Pall. of the Ranunculaceae family. There is no need to separate the paeonia into its white and red varieties. However, the *Pei yao* states, "The red paeonia is used to disperse and activate occluded blood. It is helpful in the treatment of swellings and abscesses and is used as an analgesic and menstrual-regulating agent. The white paeonia is

156

indicated for abdominal discomfort and diarrhea." It also has an anti-pyretic action and is recommended for the common cold. Thus both kinds of paeonia have similar actions in treating stagnancy of the blood, all swellings, aches, and menstrual problems. There is no significant difference between the two. There is no special processing necessary, it being cut into slices for use.

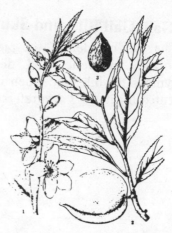

Persica 桃仁

This is the seed of *Prunus persica* (L.) Batsch of the Rosaceae family. The *Pei yao* records that it "is used to break up blood clots and move stagnation, moisten aridity, loosen bowels, and treat coughs, blood disorders, and chest pains." Thus it is indicated for diseases which involve the blood and overall pain of the body.

Before using, the coarse skin and apex of the seed are removed.

Phaseolus 赤小豆

This drug is the seed of *Phaseolus calcaratus* Roxb. of the Leguminosae family. Its functions are listed in the *Pei yao* as "a diuretic for swelling and abscesses." This indicates it has detoxifying, diuretic, and antipustulant actions.

Phellodendron 黃蘗

This is the yellow inner portion of the bark from the trunk of the *Phellodendron amurense* Rupr. of the Rutaceae family.

157

The *Pei yao* states, "It is used as an alterative,* tonic, and stomachic. Externally it is also employed as an ophthalmological and dermatological agent." That is, it has antiphlogistic, stomachic, intestinal regulatory, astringent, and antibacterial effects.

*An obsolete medical term meaning capable of restoring to health.

Pig's Gall, Gall Bile, and Skin 豬膽、豬膽汁、豬膚

The gall bladder of the pig has cholegogueous, stomachic, spasmolytic, analgesic, and detoxifying effects. Pig's gall is synonymous for bile, and when indicated, the gall bladder can be substituted for it. Pig's skin refers to the outer dermal layer.

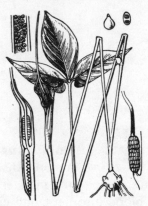

Pinellia 半夏

Pinellia is the corm of *Pinellia tuberifera* Breit. of the Araceae family. The Chinese name *pan hsia* means mid-summer and it is so named because it grows in that season. Its functions are recorded in the *Pei yao* as follows: "It is used as a sedative for cough-ups (productive cough) and vomiting with regurgitation." The former means violent coughing and the latter implies severe vomiting. Pinellia not only supresses these complaints but also dispels pathological water and renders diuresis. It also treats rising *ch'i.*

The processing methods for pinellia call for washing away the cork layer and breaking up the corm with a jujube-like kernel.

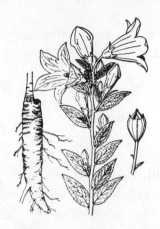

Platycodon 桔梗

This is the root of *Platycodon grandiflorum* A. DC. of the Campanulaceae family. In the *Pei yao* it says that it "is used as a stimulating expectorant for the common cold, coughs, asthma, pulmonary tuberculosis, pleuritis, etc. It is effective also in getting rid of pus and sputum.

Phytolacca 商陸根

This is the root of *Phytolacca esculenta* Van Hout. of the Phytolaccaceae family. *Pei yao* states that it "is used for edema as a diuretic." It is processed by cooking.

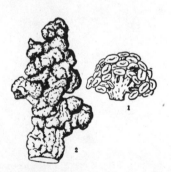

Polyporus 豬苓

This is a fungus that grows profusely on the above-ground roots of *Liquidambar formosana*. Only the core of the fungus is used medically, the crust being removed and discarded. (The fungus is of a dark color.) The *Pei yao* notes that it "moves water, dries dampness, reduces swelling, quenches thirst." In addition to being diuretic, antipyretic, and antidipsetic (thirst-quenching), polyporus also has a tranquilizing action.

159

Although most commercial products retain the crust, it is removed before use.

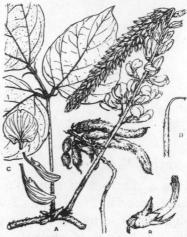

Pueraria 葛根

This is the root of *Pueraria hirsuta* Schneid. of the Leguminosae family. The *Pei yao* states that it "is used to render diaphoresis and to cleanse, cool and dissolve fever." Thus pueraria acts to promote sweating, to alleviate fever within the body, and also to relieve muscle tension in the shoulders and back, to regulate intestinal peristalsis in treating diarrhea, and to relieve tenesmus.

Rehmannia (raw) 生地黃

This drug is the rhizome of *Rehmannia glutinosa* (Gaertn.) Liobsch of the Scrophulariaceae family. Originally it was used in the raw form. However, now unless personally cultivated, it is available only in the dried or cured form in the drug store. Hence in most instances, dried rehmannia is substituted for the raw form.

Its functions as listed in the *Pei yao* are: "It is used to purge fire and cleanse heat, to stop vomiting and nosebleeds, to treat warm diarrhea, and to reduce fevers." Here the term "to purge fire" means to treat inflammations; "to cleanse heat" means to lower fever; and "warm diarrhea" refers to diarrhea with accompanying fever. In addition, rehmannia in its raw form has the effect of strengthening, nourishing, and enriching the blood. It is also hemostatic, tranquilizing, and analgesic.

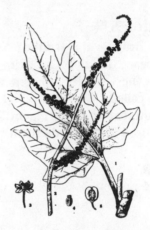

Rhubarb 大黃

Rhubarb is the rhizome of *Rheum officinale* Baill. of the Polygonaceae family. Its functions are listed in the *Pei yao* as follows "It is used exclusively as a cathartic or as a stomachic. It is helpful for dyspepsia and constipation." Rhubarb has also been reported to have an anti-inflammatory action. It is peeled and pickled in wine before use, although occasionally this process is omitted.

Sargassum (Seaweed) 海藻

This is the seaweed of *Sargassum siliquastrum* Ag. of the Alga subdivision of *Thallophyta* phylum. The *Pei yao* indicates that it "is a diuretic and is useful in treating *ying liu* (abscesses)."

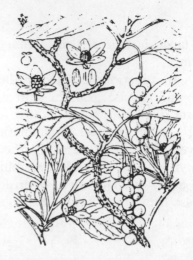

Schizandra 五味子

This drug is the fruit of *Schizandra chinensis* Baill. of the Magnoliaceae family. The skin and pulp of the fruit are sweet and bitter; the kernels, pungent and bitter; and the whole, salty. Thus it is called "five flavors." The *Pei yao* says, "It is used as an expectorant, tonic, or astringent."

It is used in the crude form without processing.

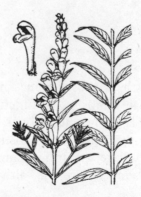

Scute 黃芩

This is the root of *Scutellaria baicalensis* Georgi of the Labiatae family. The *Pei yao* says, "It purges five and exludes dampness and is used as a clarifying, cooling, and antipyretic agent. It also has a diuretic effect." In the *Shang han lun,* whenever the prescription *hsieh-hsin-tang* is mentioned, it always contains scute.

162

Soja (Bean Relish) 香豉

Also named *tan tou shih* or simply *shih,* it is produced by salting and fermenting soya beans. A detailed description of its production may be found in Li Shih-chen's *Pen ts'ao kang mu.* Because of the superfluous and cumbersome procedure described therein, people usually use ordinary fermented soya beans and dry them.

Its medicinal efficacies as noted in the *Pei yao* indicate that it "is used to promote sweating and vomiting," which is not correct. Bean relish can be used as a digestant and it is quite nourishing. It also has antiphlogistic, antipyretic, and tranquilizing actions.

Similar to the method employed for gypsum, it is processed by wrapping in silk linen for decoction.

Tabanus (Gadfly) 䖟蟲

Tabanus is a small insect which sucks blood from animal hosts. It resembles the leech in being capable of dissolving old blood clots. The processing method consists of removing the appendages (wings and legs) and then roasting them over a fire until they are dry.

Talc 滑石

This is the naturally occurring magnesium silicate hydrate. The *Pei yao* indicates that it is used as a powder excipient, an erroneous description. Talc has the ability to eliminate urethral inflammation, mollify stimulation, and promote normal urination.

Tang-kuei 當歸

This drug is the root of *Angelica sinensis* Diels. of the Umbelliferae family. The *Pei yao* says, "It enriches and activates the blood, moistens aridity, and lubricates the intestines and is used to regulate circulation and menstruation. It is an important drug in the field of gynecology." This drug is helpful in treating anemia and is hemostatic. It warms, nourishes, enriches, and moistens the body, regulates menstruation, and has analgesic and tranquilizing properties.

163

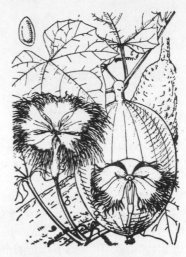

Trichosanthes Roots 栝樓根

This drug is the root of *Trichosanthes kirilowii* Max. of the Cucurbitaceae family. *Tien hua fen* is made by pulverizing the root into snow white powder.

Its functions are recorded in the *Pei yao* as "used to quench thirst, to moisten aridity, to exclude pus, to promote the growth of muscles, and to dissolve swellings." It also has a muscle-relaxing action. It is used in slices with no special processing.

Vinegar 苦酒

This is the vinegar made from rice. Its functions, as recorded in the *Pei yao,* are "to disperse extravasated blood and to dissolve carbunculous swellings and hard masses. It is also an antidote for poisoning by fish, meat, vegetables, and/or various insects."

White Bark of Tzu (raw) (*Catalpa bungei* C. A. Meyer)
生梓白皮

The origin of the plant *tzu* is not clear. In consulting Bokuya's *New Atlas of Japanese Botany* under the entry of "*Hisagi*," it states, "*Hisagi* (Chinese name *chu*) or *ihigili* (Chinese name *i*) is also named *shi* (Chinese name *tzu*). However, *tzu* is another variety of *chu.*" In Nakato Hisaken's *A Research on Ancient Medical Prescriptions,* it says that *tzu* is equivalent to *chou yao tzu shu* (literally, wine medicinal plant), and it is wrong to mistake *tzu* for *chu.* There is no such medicine by the name of *tzu pai pi* (white bark of *tzu*) on the market today. The white bark of the mulberry tree in slices is used in its place as a diuretic.

White Powder 白粉

This the powder of *Oryza sativa* L. of the Gramineae family. It has paregoric and nourishing effects. This drug is processed by roasting until a fragrance is evident, then pulverizing it into a powder.

Zanthoxylum 蜀椒

This drug has also been named Szechuan pepper. (The variety is indigenous to Szechuan, hence its name.) It is the fruit of *Zanthoxylum piperitum* DC. of the Rutaceae family. The *Pei yao* records, "It is used as an antidote, anthelmintic, and stomachic." It is also a stimulant which augments blood circulation and has stomachic, carminative, and intestine-regulating effects.

1. This book covers only a segment of the vast discipline of Chinese medicine. For instance, the herbs listed in this chapter are a few of the many sources used to make herbal medicines. For further study, please refer to the author's other works listed in the back.

Part III

Formulas of the *Shang han lun*
Key to Abbreviations of Formulas

Kuei-chih-tang 桂枝湯
(Cinnamon Combination)

3 *liang*	Cinnamon without outer bark
3 *liang*	Paeonia
3 *liang*	Licorice, seared
3 *liang*	Ginger, cut
12	Jujube, cut

Cut the first three herbs into very fine pieces. Place all the ingredients into 7 *sheng* of water and then boil down over a low flame until 3 *sheng* remain. Remove any sediment and drink 1 *sheng* while warm. Wait for a short time and then take 1 or more *sheng* of hot congee (rice gruel) to institute a joint action. Wrap the body with bedding to keep warm while perspiring freely. A simple water type of sweat is of little benefit. If the patient has perspired freely and been healed after the first dose, the remaining herb tea is not necessary. However, if sweating has not occurred, the prescription is taken as before one more time. If there is still no perspiration, an additional three doses (in shortened intervals) in about a half day's time will be required. For a serious case, the prescription should be continued for another day and night (24 hours), and the patient's condition carefully observed. Two or three daily doses (1 daily dose = 3 *sheng* in this instance) may be required for those who fail to perspire freely. Fruit, meat, noodles, garlic, onions, wine, cheese, and raw, glutinous, slippery, cold, malodorous, fatty foods are contraindicated during the treatment.

Kuei-chih-chia-ko-ken-tang 桂枝加葛根湯
(Cinnamon and Pueraria Combination)

4 *liang*	Pueraria
3 *liang*	Paeonia
3 *liang*	Ginger, cut
2 *liang*	Licorice, seared
12	Jujube, shredded
3 *liang*	Cinnamon

Place the pueraria into 1 *tou* of water and boil down until 2 *sheng* remain. Remove any white froth and add the remaining herbs. Boil again until a residual volume of 3 *sheng* remains. Remove any sediment and take 1 *sheng* of the combination while it is warm. Wrap the body with bedding to cause mild sweating. The same method of administration as employed with *Kuei-chih-tang* (Cinnamon combination) is used for this formula, i.e. the time between two doses and incompatibilities. The hot congee (rice gruel) may not be necessary.

Kuei-chih-chia-fu-tzu-tang 桂枝加附子湯
(Cinnamon, Aconite, and Jujube Combination)

3 *liang*	Cinnamon with outer bark removed
3 *liang*	Paeonia
3 *liang*	Licorice, seared
3 *liang*	Ginger, cut
12	Jujube, cut up
1	Aconite with outer bark removed and cut into eight pieces. (To remove outer bark, bake first.)

Place the herbs in 7 *sheng* of water. Boil down to 3 *sheng*, remove the sediment, and drink 1 *sheng* of the combination while warm. For administration and dosing regimen follow the instructions given for *Kuei-chih-tang* (Cinnamon Combination).

Kuei-chih-chu-shao-yao-tang 桂枝去芍藥湯
(Cinnamon minus Paeonia Combination)

3 *liang*	Cinnamon without outer bark
2 *liang*	Licorice, seared
3 *liang*	Ginger, cut
12	Jujube, broken into small pieces

Place the above four items in 7 *sheng* of water. Boil down until 3 *sheng* remain, and then take 1 *sheng* of the prescription while warm. The administration and dosing regimen are the same as for *Kuei-chih-tang* (Cinnamon Combination).

Kuei-chih-chu-shao-yao-chia-fu-tzu-tang
桂枝去芍藥加附子湯
(Cinnamon, Ginger, and Aconite Combination)

3 *liang*	Cinnamon with outer bark removed
2 *liang*	Licorice, seared
3 *liang*	Ginger, cut
12	Jujube
1	Aconite heated to remove outer bark and cut into 8 pieces

Place the five herbs in 7 *sheng* of water. Boil down until 3 *sheng* remain, remove the sediment, and take 1 *sheng* of the combination while warm. Follow the regimen for *Kuei-chih-tang* (Cinnamon Combination) for administration and dosing.

Kuei-chih-ma-huang-ko-pan-tang 桂枝麻黃各半湯
(Cinnamon and Ma-huang Combination)

1 *liang* 16 *chu*	Cinnamon with outer bark removed
1 *liang*	Paeonia
1 *liang*	Ginger, cut
1 *liang*	Licorice, seared
1 *liang*	*Ma-huang* without nodes
4	Jujube, broken into small pieces
24	Apricot seed, soaked to remove outer skin and apexes; twin kernels also removed

Place 1 *liang* of *ma-huang* in 5 *sheng* of water. Boil and remove the white froth before adding the other herbs. Boil again down to a residual 1 *sheng* 8 *ho*; remove the sediment and take 6 *ho* of the combination while warm. For administration and dosing regimen, follow the rules given for *Kuei-chih-tang* (Cinnamon Combination).

Kuei-chih-erh-ma-huang-i-tang 桂枝二麻黃一湯
(Ma-huang and Double Cinnamon Combination)

1 *liang* 17 *chu* Cinnamon with outer bark removed

1 *liang* 6 *chu* Paeonia
16 *chu* *Ma-huang* without nodes
1 *liang* 6 *chu* Ginger, cut
16   Apricot seed without outer skin and apexes
2 *liang* 2 *chu* Licorice, seared
5   Jujube, shredded

Place the *ma-huang* in 5 *sheng* of water. Boil and remove the floating white froth; then add the other herbs. Boil again until 2 *sheng* remain. Remove any sediment and take 1 *sheng* of the combination while warm. The administration and dosing regimen follows that of *Kuei-chih-tang* (Cinnamon Combination).

Pai-hu-chia-jen-sheng-tang 白虎加人参湯
(Ginseng and Gypsum Combination)

6 *liang* Anemarrhena
1 *chin* Gypsum, pulverized and wrapped up in silk cloth
2 *liang* Licorice, seared
6 *ho* Oryza
3 *liang* Ginseng

Place the five herbs in 1 *tou* of water and boil until the oryza is well cooked. Remove the sediment and take 1 *sheng* of the combination while warm. This is taken three times daily.

Kuei-chih-erh-yueh-pei-i-tang 桂枝二越婢一湯
(Cinnamon, Ma-huang, and Gypsum Combination)

18 *chu* Cinnamon with outer bark removed
18 *chu* Paeonia
18 *chu* *Ma-huang*
18 *chu* Licorice, seared
4   Jujube, shredded
1 *liang* 2 *chu* Ginseng, cut
24 *chu* Gypsum, ground and wrapped in silk cloth

Place the *ma-huang* in 5 *sheng* of water. Boil and remove the floating froth before adding the other herbs. Boil again until only 2 *sheng* remain. Remove the sediment and take 1 *sheng* of the combination while warm.

Kuei-chih-chu-kuei-chia-fu-ling-pai-chu-tang

桂枝去桂加茯苓白朮湯

(Hoelen, Atractylodes, and Paeonia Combination)

3 *liang*	Paeonia
2 *liang*	Licorice, seared
3 *liang*	Ginger, cut
3 *liang*	Atractylodes
3 *liang*	Hoelen
12	Jujube, shredded

Place the above herbs in 8 *sheng* of water. Boil the mixture down to 3 *sheng* and remove the sediment. Take 1 *sheng* of the prescription while warm. If diuresis occurs, the condition is relieved.

Kan-tsao-kan-chiang-tang 甘草乾薑湯
(Licorice and Ginger Combination)

4 *liang*	Licorice, seared
2 *liang*	Ginger

Place the two herbs in 3 *sheng* of water. Boil until only 1 *sheng* 5 *ho* remain and then remove any sediment. Divide the prescription into two doses and take while warm.

Tiao-wei-cheng-chi-tang 調胃承氣湯
(Rhubarb and Mirabilitum Combination)

4 *liang*	Rhubarb with outer bark removed and washed with clear wine
2 *liang*	Licorice, seared
½ *sheng*	Mirabilitum

171

Place the first two herbs in 3 *sheng* of water and boil until 1 *sheng* remains. Remove any sediment and then add the mirabilitum. Boil again over a low flame and then sip the prescription while it is warm.

Szu-ni-tang 四逆湯
(Aconite, Ginger, and Licorice Combination)

2 *liang*	Licorice, seared
1½ *liang*	Ginger
1	Aconite, raw with outer bark removed and then cut into eight pieces.

Place the above herbs in 3 *sheng* of water. Boil over a low flame until only 1 *sheng* 2 *ho* remain. Remove sediment and take the combination in two separate doses while warm.

Ko-ken-tang 葛根湯
(Pueraria Combination)

4 *liang*	Pueraria
3 *liang*	*Ma-huang* without nodes
2 *liang*	Cinnamon without outer bark
3 *liang*	Ginger, cut
2 *liang*	Licorice, seared
2 *liang*	Paeonia
12	Jujube, shredded

Place the first two herbs in 1 *tou* of water. Boil down to 8 *sheng* and remove the white foam before adding the other herbs. Boil again until only 3 *sheng* remain. Remove the sediment and take 1 *sheng* of the combination while warm. Then wrap the body with bedding to keep warm and to cause mild sweating. The administration, dosing regimen and incompatibilities are the same as for *Kuei-chih-tang* (Cinnamon Combination).

Ko-ken-chia-pan-hsia-tang 葛根加半夏湯
(Pueraria and Pinellia Combination)

4 *liang*	Pueraria
3 *liang*	*Ma-huang* without nodes
2 *liang*	Licorice, seared
2 *liang*	Paeonia
2 *liang*	Cinnamon with outer bark removed
3 *liang*	Ginger, cut
½ *sheng*	Pinellia, washed
12	Jujube, shredded

Place the first two herbs in 1 *tou* of water. Boil the mixture down to 8 *sheng*. Remove the floating froth and then add the rest of the herbs. Reboil the contents until 3 *sheng* remain. Remove any sediment and take 1 *sheng* of the combination while it is warm. Then cover the body with blankets to keep warm and to cause mild sweating.

Ko-ken-huang-lien-huang-chin-kan-tsao-tang
葛根黃連黃芩甘草湯

(L. S. C. and Pueraria Combination)

½ *chin*	Pueraria
2 *liang*	Licorice, seared
3 *liang*	Scute
3 *liang*	Coptis

Place the pueraria in 8 *sheng* of water and boil the mixture until 6 *sheng* remain. Then add the other herbs. Boil again until only 2 *sheng* are left. Remove any sediment. Divide the remainder into two doses and take while warm.

Ma-huang-tang 麻黃湯
(Ma-huang Combination)

3 *liang*	*Ma-huang* without nodes
2 *liang*	Cinnamon without outer bark

1 *liang*   Licorice, seared
70 pieces Apricot seed with outer skin and apexes removed

At first put the *ma-huang* in 9 *sheng* of water and boil until the mixture is reduced to 7 *sheng*. Remove the floating white foam before adding the rest of the herbs. Continue boiling the mixture until there remains but 2½ *sheng*. Remove the residue and then take 8 *ho* of the combination while it is warm. Then wrap the body in bedding to keep warm. If mild perspiring results, hot congee (rice gruel) is not necessary. Depending upon the severity and amount of perspiration achieved, the administration and dosage of the prescription is the same as for *Kuei-chih-tang* (Cinnamon Combination).

Ta-ching-lung-tang 大靑龍湯
(Major Blue Dragon Combination)

6 *liang*   *Ma-huang* without nodes
2 *liang*   Cinnamon with outer bark removed
2 *liang*   Licorice, seared
40 pieces Apricot seed with outer skin and apexes removed
3 *liang*   Ginger, cut up
10   Jujube, shredded
1 "egg"   Gypsum, ground and wrapped in silk cloth

Place the first herb in 9 *sheng* of water. Boil the mixture until only 7 *sheng* remain. Remove the floating froth and add the other herbs. Boil the contents down to 3 *sheng* and remove any sediment. Take 1 *sheng* of the combination while it is warm. Wrap the body in blankets to keep warm and to cause mild perspiring. If the patient has adequately perspired and feels better after one dosage, the remaining herb tea is not necessary.

Hsiao-ching-lung-tang 小靑龍湯
(Minor Blue Dragon Combination)

3 *liang*   *Ma-huang* without nodes
3 *liang*   Paeonia

174

3 *liang*   Asarum
3 *liang*   Ginger
3 *liang*   Licorice, seared
3 *liang*   Cinnamon with outer bark removed
½ *chin*   Schizandra
½ *shen*   Pinellia, washed

At first, place the *ma-huang* in 1 *tou* of water. Boil down to 8 *sheng* and remove the white froth before adding the other herbs. Then boil until only 3 *sheng* remain. Strain and take 1 *sheng* while warm.

Kuei-chih-chia-hou-pu-hsing-tzu-tang 桂枝加厚朴杏子湯
(M.A. and Cinnamon Combination)

3 *liang*   Cinnamon with outer bark removed
2 *liang*   Licorice, seared
3 *liang*   Ginger, cut
3 *liang*   Paeonia
12   Jujube, shredded
2 *liang*   Magnolia, seared with outer bark removed
50   Apricot seed with outer skin and apexes removed.

Place the above herbs in 7 *sheng* of water. Simmer them over a low flame until only 3 *sheng* remain. Strain and take 1 *sheng* while warm. Then wrap the body in bedding to keep warm and to cause mild sweating.

Kuei-chih-chia-shao-yao-sheng-chiang-ko-i-liang-jen-sheng-san-liang-hsin-chia-tang
桂枝加芍藥生薑各一兩人參三兩新加湯
(Cinnamon, Paeonia, Ginger, and Ginseng Combination)

3 *liang*   Cinnamon with outer bark removed
4 *liang*   Paeonia
2 *liang*   Licorice, seared
3 *liang*   Ginseng
12   Jujube
4 *liang*   Ginger

175

Place the six herbs in 1 *tou* 2 *sheng* of water. Boil down until only 3 *sheng* remain. Remove any sediment and take 1 *sheng* of the decoction while warm.

Ma-huang-hsing-jen-kan-tsao-shih-kao-tang
麻黃杏仁甘草石膏湯

(Apricot Seed and Ma-huang Combination)

4 *liang*	*Ma-huang* without nodes
50	Apricot seed with outer skin and apexes removed
2 *liang*	Licorice, seared
½ *chin*	Gypsum ground and wrapped in silk cloth

At first place the *ma-huang* in 7 *sheng* of water. Boil down to 5 *sheng*. Remove the white froth and then add the other herbs. Reboil until only 2 *sheng* remain. Remove any sediment and take 1 *sheng* while warm.

Kuei-chih-kan-tsao-tang 桂枝甘草湯
(Cinnamon and Licorice Combination)

4 *liang*	Cinnamon with outer bark removed
2 *liang*	Licorice seared

Place the above herbs in 3 *sheng* of water. Boil the mixture down to 1 *sheng*. Remove the sediment and take the combination while warm.

Fu-ling-kuei-chih-kan-tsao-ta-tsao-tang
茯苓桂枝甘草大棗湯

(C. L. J. and Hoelen Combination)

½ *chin*	Hoelen
4 *liang*	Cinnamon with outer bark removed
2 *liang*	Licorice, seared
15	Ginger, Shredded

At first place the hoelen into 1 *tou* of throughly stirred (aerated) water. Boil the mixture down to 8 *sheng* and then add the remaining herbs. Boil again until 3 *sheng* remain. Strain and then take 1 *sheng* warmed three times during the day.

Hou-pu-sheng-chiang-pan-hsia-kan-tsao-jen-sheng-tang
厚朴生薑半夏甘草人參湯
(Magnolia Five Combination)

½ *chin*	Magnolia, seared with outer bark removed
½ *chin*	Ginger, cut
½ *shen*	Pinellia, washed
2 *liang*	Licorice, seared
1 *liang*	Ginseng

Place the above herbs in 1 *tou* of water. Boil until only 3 *sheng* remain. Remove the residue. Take 1 *sheng* of the combination warmed three times during the day.

Fu-ling-kuei-chih-pai-chu-kan-tsao-tang
茯苓桂枝白朮甘草湯
(Hoelen, Licorice, and Atractylodes Combination)

4 *liang*	Hoelen
3 *liang*	Cinnamon with outer bark removed
2 *liang*	Atractylodes, seared
2 *liang*	Licorice, seared

Place the above four herbs in 6 *sheng* of water. Boil down until only 3 *sheng* remain and remove all sediment. Take the combination warmed three times during the day.

Shao-yao-kan-tsao-fu-tzu-tang 芍藥甘草附子湯
(Paeonia, Licorice, and Aconite Combination)

3 *liang*	Paeonia
3 *liang*	Licorice, seared
1	Aconite with outer bark removed, baked, and cut into eight pieces.

Place the above herbs in 5 *sheng* of water. Boil until only 1 *sheng* 5 *ho* remain. Strain to remove sediment and take the combination warmed three times during the day.

Fu-ling-szu-ni-tang 茯苓四逆湯
(Hoelen, Licorice, Aconite, and Ginseng Combination)

4 *liang*	Hoelen
1 *liang*	Ginseng
1	Aconite, raw, with outer bark removed and cut into eight pieces
2 *liang*	Licorice, seared
1½ *liang*	Ginger

Place the five herbs into 5 *sheng* of water. Boil them until only 3 *sheng* is left. Remove the sediment. Take 7 *ho* warmed three times during the day.

Wu-ling-san 五苓散
(Hoelen Five Herb Formula)

18 *chu*	Polyporus with outer bark removed
1 *liang* 6 *chu*	Alisma
18 *chu*	Atractylodes
18 *chu*	Hoelen
½ *liang*	Cinnamon with outer bark removed

Pound the above herbs into a powder. Take 2 grams with rice soup three times daily. The patient should drink warm water frequently during treatment to cause sweating which in turn instigates recovery.

Fu-ling-kan-tsao-tang 茯苓甘草湯
(Hoelen and Licorice Combination)

2 *liang*	Hoelen
2 *liang*	Cinnamon with outer bark removed

178

1 *liang*   Licorice, seared
3 *liang*   Ginger, cut

Place the above herbs in 4 *sheng* of water. Boil down to 2 *sheng* and remove the sediment. Take the combination warmed three times during the day.

Chih-tzu-shih-tang 梔子豉湯
(Gardenia and Soja Combination)

14   Gardenia, cut up
2 *liang*   Licorice, seared
4 *ho*   Soja, wrapped in silk cloth

Place the first two herbs in 4 *sheng* of water and boil them until 2½ *sheng* are left. Then add the third herb and boil down until only 1½ *sheng* remain. Remove the sediment and take one half of the decoction while warm. Should vomiting occur, the remaining herb tea should not be taken.

Chih-tzu-sheng-chiang-shih-tang 梔子生薑豉湯
(Gardenia, Ginger, and Soja Combination)

14   Gardenia, cut up
5 *liang*   Ginger
4 *ho*   Soja, wrapped in silk cloth

Place the first two herbs in 4 *sheng* of water and boil down to 2½ *sheng*. Place the third herb in this mixture. Boil again until only 1½ *sheng* remain. Remove any residue and take one-half of the combination while warm. If vomiting occurs, do not take the remaining herb tea.

Chih-tzu-hou-pu-tang 梔子厚朴湯
(Gardenia and Magnolia Combination)

14   Gardenia, cut up

4 *liang*   Magnolia, with outer bark removed and seared.

4   *Chih-shih,* dipped and seared until yellow

Place the above herbs in 3½ *sheng* of water. Boil the mixture until only 1½ *sheng* remain. Remove the residue and take one half of the decoction while warm. If vomiting occurs, do not take the remaining herb tea.

Chih-tzu-kan-chiang-tang 栀子乾薑湯
(Gardenia and Ginger Combination)

14   Gardenia, cut up
1 *liang*   Ginger

Place the two herbs in 3½ *sheng* of water and boil down to 1½ *sheng.* Strain and take one half of the amount while warm. If vomiting occurs, do not take the remaining herb tea.

Kan-chiang-fu-tzu-tang 乾薑附子湯
(Ginger and Aconite Combination)

1 *liang*   Ginger
1   Aconite, raw, with outer bark removed and cut into eight pieces

Place the above herbs in 3 *sheng* of water. Boil the mixture down until only 1 *sheng* remains. Strain and take the combination while warm.

Hsiao-chai-hu-tang 小柴胡湯
(Minor Bupleurum Combination)

½ *chin*   Bupleurum
3 *liang*   Scute
3 *liang*   Ginseng
½ *sheng* Pinellia
3 *liang*   Licorice, seared

3 *liang*   Ginger, cut
12   Jujube, shredded

Put the above herbs in 1 *tou* 2 *sheng* of water. Boil them until only 6 *sheng* remain. Remove the sediment; then boil again down to 3 *sheng*. Take 1 *sheng* of this mixture warmed, three times daily.

Hsiao-chien-chung-tang 小建中湯
(Minor Cinnamon and Paeonia Combination)

3 *liang*   Cinnamon with outer bark removed
2 *liang*   Licorice, seared
12   Jujube, shredded
6 *liang*   Paeonia
3 *liang*   Ginger, cut
1 *sheng*   Maltose

Place the first five herbs in 7 *sheng* of water. Boil the mixture down until only 3 *sheng* remain. Remove the residue and add the maltose. Simmer over a low flame until the latter is completely dissolved and then take 1 *sheng* of the combination warmed three times daily.

Ta-chai-hu-tang 大柴胡湯
(Major Bupleurum Combination)

½ *chin*   Bupleurum
3 *liang*   Scute
3 *liang*   Paeonia
½ *sheng*   Pinellia, washed
5 *liang*   Ginger, cut
4   *Chih-shih*, seared
12   Jujube, shredded
2 *liang*   Rhubarb

Place the above herbs in 1 *tou* 2 *sheng* of water. Boil until only 6 *sheng* are left and remove the sediment. Then boil again until only 3 *sheng* remain. Take 1 *sheng* of this mixture warmed three times daily.

Chai-hu-chia-mang-hsiao-tang 柴胡加芒硝湯
(Bupleurum and Mirabilitum Combination)

2 *liang* 16 *chu*	Bupleurum
1 *liang*	Scute
2 *liang*	Ginseng
1 *liang*	Licorice, seared
1 *liang*	Ginger, cut
20 *chu*	Pinellia washed
4	Jujube, shredded
2 *liang*	Mirabilitum

Place the first seven herbs in 4 *sheng* of water and boil down until only 2 *sheng* remain. Remove the sediment and reboil the mixture after adding the mirabilitum. Take the combination warmed in two doses.

Tao-ho-cheng-chi-tang 桃核承氣湯
(Persica and Rhubarb Combination)

50	Persica with outer skin and apexes removed
4 *liang*	Rhubarb
2 *liang*	Cinnamon with outer bark removed
2 *liang*	Licorice, seared
2 *liang*	Mirabilitum

Place the first four herbs in 7 *sheng* of water. Boil them until the amount is reduced to 2½ *sheng*. Remove the sediment and add the mirabilitum. Simmer the mixture over a low flame. Take 5 *ho* of the combination warmed three times daily.

Chai-hu-chia-lung-ku-mu-li-tang 柴胡加龍骨牡蠣湯
(Bupleurum and Dragon Bone Combination)

4 *liang*	Bupleurum
1½ *liang*	Dragon bone
1½ *liang*	Scute
1½ *liang*	Ginger, cut
1½ *liang*	Minium
1½ *liang*	Ginseng
1½ *liang*	Cinnamon with outer bark removed
1½ *liang*	Hoelen
2½ *ho*	Pinellia washed
2 *liang*	Rhubarb, cut into dices
1½ *liang*	Oyster shell, simmered
6	Jujube, shredded

Place the first eleven herbs into 8 *sheng* of water. Boil the contents down to 4 *sheng* and then add the rhubarb. Reboil the mixture, skim the residue, and take 1 *sheng* of the combination while warm.

Kuei-chih-chu-shao-yao-chia-shu-chi-mu-li-lung-ku-chiu-ni-tang 桂枝去芍藥加蜀漆牡蠣龍骨救逆湯
(Cinnamon, Dichroa, Oyster Shell, and Dragon Bone Combination)

3 *liang*	Cinnamon with outer bark removed
2 *liang*	Licorice, seared
3 *liang*	Ginger, cut
12	Jujube, shredded
5 *liang*	Oyster shell, simmered
3 *liang*	Dichroa, washed until free from fishy odor
4 *liang*	Dragon bone

First place the dichroa in 1 *tou* 2 *sheng* of water. Boil this mixture down to 1 *tou*; then add the remaining herbs. Boil again down to 3 *sheng*. Remove any sediment and take 1 *sheng* of this prescription while warm.

Kuei-chih-chia-kuei-tang 桂枝加桂湯
(Cinnamon, Licorice, and Ginger Combination)

5 *liang*	Cinnamon with outer bark removed
3 *liang*	Paeonia
3 *liang*	Ginger, cut
2 *liang*	Licorice, seared
12	Jujube, shredded

Place the above herbs into 7 *sheng* of water. Boil the mixture down to 3 *sheng* and remove the residue. Take 1 *sheng* of the combination while warm.

Kuei-chih-kan-tsao-lung-ku-mu-li-tang
桂枝甘草龍骨牡蠣湯
(Cinnamon, Licorice, Oyster Shell, and Dragon Bone Combination)

1 *liang*	Cinnamon with outer bark removed
2 *liang*	Licorice, seared
2 *liang*	Oyster shell, simmered
2 *liang*	Dragon bone

Place the above four herbs in 5 *sheng* of water. Boil until the mixture is reduced to 2½ *sheng* and strain. Take 8 *ho* of this prescription warmed three times daily.

Ti-tang-tang 抵當湯
(Rhubarb and Leech Combination)

13	Leech, simmered
13	Tabanus with wings and feet removed and simmered
20	Persica with outer skin and apexes removed
3 *liang*	Rhubarb, washed in wine

Place the above herbs in 5 *sheng* of water. Reduce the contents to 3 *sheng* by boiling. Remove the sediment and take 1 *sheng* of the mixture while warm. If there is no discharge of blood, continue taking the prescription.

Ti-tang-wan 抵當丸
(Rhubarb and Leech Formula)

20	Leech, simmered
20	Tabanus with wings and feet removed and simmered
25	Persica with outer skin and apexes removed
3 *liang*	Rhubarb, washed in wine

Grind the above ingredients together and make into 4 pills. Place one pill in 1 *sheng* of water and boil until 7 *ho* remain; then take the decoction. One day later, blood will be discharged.

Ta-hsien-hsiung-wan 大陷胸丸
(Major Rhubarb and Mirabilitum Formula)

½ *chin*	Rhubarb
½ *sheng*	Lepidium, simmered
½ *sheng*	Mirabilitum
½ *sheng*	Apricot Seed with outer bark and apexes removed, simmered until black.

Grind the first two herbs into powder and sift them. Pound the other two herbs into a lard-like semi-solid and then mix in the powder; form into bullet-like pills. Meanwhile grind 1.7 *chien* (1 *chien* = 0.1 *liang*) of *kan-sui* into powder and then put it together with one of the pills previously prepared in 2 *ho* of mel and 2 *sheng* of water. Boil until the contents are reduced to 1 *sheng*. Take this prescription all at once while warm. Diarrhea should result overnight. If not, one dose at a time should follow until diarrhea occurs. This formula should be carefully prepared according to the instructions.

Ta-hsien-hsiung-tang 大陷胸湯
(Rhubarb and Kan-sui Combination)

6 *liang*	Rhubarb with outer bark removed
1 *sheng*	Mirabilitum
1 *chien*	*Kan-sui*, pulverized

185

Place the rhubarb in 6 *sheng* of water. Boil the mixture down to 2 *sheng* and remove the sediment. Then add the mirabilitum and reboil for just a little while. Finally, augment the combination with the powder of *kan-sui* while boiling. Take 1 *sheng* of the combination while warm. If diarrhea occurs, no further herb tea is needed.

Hsiao-hsien-hsiung-tang 小陷胸湯
(Minor Trichosanthes Combination)

1 *liang*	Coptis
½ *sheng*	Pinellia, washed
1	Trichosanthes, a large one

Place the trichosanthes in 6 *sheng* of water. Boil the contents until 3 *sheng* remains. Remove the sediment and add the other two herbs. Boil the mixture down to 2 *sheng*. Once again remove the sediment and take the prescription warmed three times during the day.

Wen-ke-san 文蛤散
(Meretrix Formula)

| 5 *liang* | Meretrix |

Grind the herb into powder. Take 2.0 grams of the powder together with 5 *ho* of boiled warm water.

Chieh-keng-pai-san (San-wu-hsiao-pai-san) 桔梗白散
(Platycodon and Croton Formula)

3 *fen*	Platycodon
1 *fen*	Croton with outer coat and center core removed, simmered until black, and pounded into a semi-solid state
3 *fen*	Fritillaria

186

Grind the above herbs into powder; then mix and pound well in a mortar. Take with rice congee (gruel). Strong patients can take 0.5 grams of the prescription in a single dose, whereas weaker individuals must be given a smaller amount. Vomiting occurs when the disease is above the diaphragm and diarrhea when the disease is below it. If there is no diarrhea, take one glass of hot congee. One glass of cold congee should be taken if prolonged diarrhea is present. (Hot congee enhances the carthartic action of this formula and cold congee inhibits it.)

Chai-hu-kuei-chih-tang 柴胡桂枝湯
(Bupleurum and Cinnamon Combination)

1½ *liang*	Cinnamon with outer bark removed
1½ *liang*	Scute
1½ *liang*	Ginseng
1 *liang*	Licorice, seared
2.5 *ho*	Pinellia, washed
1½ *liang*	Paeonia
6	Jujube, shredded
1½ *liang*	Ginger, cut
4 *liang*	Bupleurum

Place the above herbs in 7 *sheng* of water and boil until the contents measures 3 *sheng*. Remove the sediment and take 1 *sheng* of the prescription while warm.

Chai-hu-kuei-chih-kan-chiang-tang 柴胡桂枝乾薑湯
(Bupleurum, Cinnamon, and Ginger Combination)

½ *chin*	Bupleurum
3 *liang*	Cinnamon with outer bark removed
2 *liang*	Ginger
4 *liang*	Trichosanthes
3 *liang*	Scute
2 *liang*	Oyster shell, simmered
2 *liang*	Licorice, Seared

187

Place the above herbs in 12 *sheng* of water and boil until the contents is reduced to 6 *sheng*. Remove the residue and reboil to a concentration of 3 *sheng*. Take 1 *sheng* of the prescription while warm three times daily. The first dose may cause a slight reaction but succeeding portions should result in sweating which is necessary for recovery.

Pan-hsia-hsieh-hsin-tang 半夏瀉心湯
(Pinellia Combination)

½ *sheng*	Pinellia, washed
3 *liang*	Scute, seared
3 *liang*	Ginger, seared
3 *liang*	Ginseng, seared
3 *liang*	Licorice, seared
1 *liang*	Coptis
12	Jujube, shredded

Place the seven herbs in 1 *tou* of water and boil down until 6 *sheng* remain. Remove the sediment and reduce the contents to 3 *sheng* by reboiling. Take 1 *sheng* of the combination warmed three times daily.

Shih-tsao-tang 十棗湯
(Jujube Combination)

	Genkwa
Equal parts	*Kan-sui*
	Euphorbia
10	Jujube, shredded

Pulverize equal parts of the first three herbs separately into powders. Place 10 large jujube in 1½ *sheng* of water. Reduce the contents to 8 *ho* by boiling and remove the residue; then add the above powders. Strong individuals can take 1 gram of the powder for a single dose whereas the delicately constituted may take only a half portion warmed. If there is little diarrhea and healing is not complete, a second dose must be taken the next day. Once diarrhea

188

is induced, rice congee should be taken to strengthen the body.

Ta-huang-huang-lien-hsieh-hsin-tang 大黃黃連瀉心湯
(Rhubarb, Coptis, and Scute Combination)

2 *liang*	Rhubarb
1 *liang*	Coptis
*1 *liang*	Scute

*This herb is not included in the formula in the original text. However, some scholars such as Lin I, Asada Sohaku, etc. rebuked the formula and verified from investigation that this formula should contain this herb because most other *Hsieh-hsing-tangs* do.

Place the above herbs in 2 *sheng* of thoroughly boiled water and soak for awhile. Strain to remove the residue, divide the prescription into two doses, and take while warm.

Fu-tzu-hsieh-hsin-tang 附子瀉心湯
(Rhubarb and Aconite Combination)

2 *liang*	Rhubarb
1 *liang*	Coptis
1 *liang*	Scute
2	Aconite, baked to remove bark, boiled, and then the juice extracted

Cut the first three herbs into pieces and stir into 2 *sheng* of thoroughly boiled water. Soak for a while, strain to remove the sediment, and then add the juice of aconite. Divide the combination into two doses and take warmed.

Sheng-chiang-hsieh-hsin-tang 生薑瀉心湯
(Pinellia and Ginger Combination)

4 *liang*	Ginger, cut
3 *liang*	Licorice, seared
3 *liang*	Ginseng

189

1 *liang*   Ginger (dried)
3 *liang*   Scute
½ *sheng* Pinellia, washed
1 *liang*   Coptis
12   Jujube, shredded

Place the above herbs in 1 *tou* of water. Reduce the contents to 6 *sheng* by boiling and strain. Reboil until only 3 *sheng* remain. Take 1 *sheng* of the prescription three times daily.

Kan-tsao-hsieh-hsin-tang 甘草瀉心湯
(Licorice and Pinellia Combination)

4 *liang*   Licorice, seared
3 *liang*   Scute
3 *liang*   Ginger
3 *liang*   Ginseng
½ *sheng* Pinellia, washed
12   Jujube, shredded
1 *liang*   Coptis

Place the above herbs in 1 *tou* of water. Boil the mixture down to 6 *sheng* and remove the sediment. Reduce the contents to 3 *sheng* by reboiling. Take 1 *sheng* of the formula warmed three times daily.

Chih-shih-chih-yu-yu-liang-tang 赤石脂禹餘糧湯
(Kaolin and Limonite Combination)

1 *chin*   Kaolin, broken into pieces
1 *chin*   Limonite, broken into pieces

Place the above herbs in 6 *sheng* of water. Reduce the contents to 2 *sheng* by boiling. Remove the residue and take the prescription warmed three times daily.

190

Hsuan-fu-hua-tai-che-shih-tang 旋覆花代赭石湯
(Inula and Hematite Combination)

3 *liang*	Inula
2 *liang*	Ginseng
5 *liang*	Ginger
1 *liang*	Hematite
3 *liang*	Licorice, seared
½ *chin*	Pinellia, washed
12	Jujube, shredded

Put all seven herbs in 1 *tou* of water and boil the contents down to 6 *sheng*. Strain, and then boil further until the amount remaining is 3 *sheng*. Take 1 *sheng* of the formula warmed three times daily.

Kuei-chih-jen-sheng-tang 桂枝人参湯
(Cinnamon and Ginseng Combination)

4 *liang*	Cinnamon with outer bark removed
4 *liang*	Licorice, seared
3 *liang*	Atractylodes
3 *liang*	Ginseng
3 *liang*	Ginger

Place the last four herbs in 9 *sheng* of water and boil until only 5 *sheng* remain. Add the cinnamon and reduce the contents to 3 *sheng* by reboiling. Remove the residue and take 1 *sheng* of the combination while warm.

Kua-ti-san 瓜蒂散
(Melon Pedicle Formula)

1 *fen*	Melon pedicle, simmered until yellow
1 *fen*	Phaseolus

Pound the above herbs into powder and then sift them separately. Combine the two herbs and measure out 1 *chien* of the powder combination. Place 1 *ho* of soja in 7 *ho* of hot water and boil into a putty gruel. Remove the sediment and stir in the above powder. The mixture should be taken while warm. If no vomiting ensues, gradually increase the dose until it is induced.

Huang-chin-tang 黃芩湯
(Scute Combination)

3 *liang*	Scute
2 *liang*	Paeonia
2 *liang*	Licorice, seared
12	Jujube, shredded

Place the above herbs in one *tou* of water and boil down to 3 *sheng*. Strain and take 1 *sheng* of the formula while warm.

Huang-chin-chia-pan-hsia-sheng-chiang-tang

黃芩加半夏生薑湯

(Scute, Pinellia, and Ginger Combination)

3 *liang*	Scute
2 *liang*	Paeonia
2 *liang*	Licorice, seared
12	Jujube, shredded
½ *sheng*	Pinellia, washed
1½ *liang*	Ginger, cut

Place the six herbs in 1 *tou* of water and boil down to 3 *sheng*. Strain and take 1 *sheng* of the prescription while warm.

Huang-lien-tang 黃連湯
(Coptis Combination)

3 *liang*	Coptis
3 *liang*	Licorice, seared
3 *liang*	Ginger
3 *liang*	Cinnamon with outer bark removed
2 *liang*	Ginseng
½ *sheng*	Pinellia, washed

12   Jujube, shredded

Place the above herbs in 1 *tou* of water and boil until the contents is reduced to 6 *sheng*. Remove the sediment and take the formula while warm.

Kuei-chih-fu-tzu-tang 桂枝附子湯
(Cinnamon and Aconite Combination)

4 *liang*   Cinnamon with outer bark removed
3   Aconite, baked with outer bark removed; then cut into eight pieces
3 *liang*   Ginger, cut
12   Jujube, shredded
2 *liang*   Licorice, seared

Place the above herbs in 6 *sheng* of water and boil until only 2 *sheng* remain. Strain and take the combination in three separate doses while warm.

Chu-kuei-chia-pai-chu-tang 去桂加白朮湯
(Aconite and Atractylodes Combination)

3   Aconite, baked with outer bark removed, then shredded
4 *liang*   Atractylodes
3 *liang*   Ginger, cut
2 *liang*   Licorice, seared
12   Jujube, shredded

Place the five herbs in 6 *sheng* of water and boil until 2 *sheng* remain. Remove the residue and take the combination warmed in three doses. The patient will notice a generalized numbness after the first dose. Continue the prescription for a second and third time at half-day intervals. A sensation of pressure in the head is no cause for alarm as it signifies the aconite and atractylodes are acting to dispel the dampness beneath the skin.

193

Kan-tsao-fu-tzu-tang 甘草附子湯
(Licorice and Aconite Combination)

2 *liang*	Licorice, seared
2	Aconite, baked to remove the outer bark
2 *liang*	Atractylodes
4 *liang*	Cinnamon with outer bark removed

Put the four herbs in 6 *sheng* of water and boil until the amount is reduced to 3 *sheng*. Remove the residue and take 1 *sheng* of the prescription three times daily warmed.

Pai-hu-tang 白虎湯
(Gypsum Combination)

6 *liang*	Anemarrhena
1 *chin*	Gypsum, ground
2 *liang*	Licorice, seared
6 *ho*	Oryza

Place the four herbs in 1 *tou* of water and boil the mixture until the oryza is well cooked. Strain off the sediment and take 1 *sheng* of the formula three times daily.

Chih-kan-tsao-tang 炙甘草湯
(Baked Licorice Combination)

4 *liang*	Licorice seared
3 *liang*	Ginger, cut
2 *liang*	Ginseng
1 *chin*	Rehmannia
3 *liang*	Cinnamon with outer bark removed
2 *liang*	Gelatin
½ *sheng*	Ophiopogon, decored
½ *sheng*	Linum
30	Jujube, shredded

Except for the gelatin, put the above herbs into a mixture of

194

7 *sheng* of wine and 8 *sheng* of water. Boil the mixture until only 3 *sheng* remain. Strain and then add the gelatin. Boil again until the latter is well dissolved. Take 1 *sheng* of the combination three times daily.

Ta-cheng-chi-tang 大承氣湯
(Major Rhubarb Combination)

4 *liang*	Rhubarb
½ *chin*	Magnolia, seared with outer bark removed
5	*Chih-shih*, seared
3 *ho*	Mirabilitum

Place the magnolia and *chih-shih* in 1 *tou* of water and reduce and volume to 5 *sheng* by boiling. Remove the sediment and then add the rhubarb . Boil further until there remain only 2 *sheng*. Skim off the residue, add the mirabilitum to the mixture, and reboil for a short time. Take the prescription while warm.

Hsiao-cheng-chi-tang 小承氣湯
(Minor Rhubarb Combination)

4 *liang*	Rhubarb
2 *liang*	Magnolia, seared with outer bark removed
3	*Chih-shih*, seared

Place the above herbs in 4 *sheng* of water and boil down until only 1 *sheng* remains. Strain and take the combination in two separate doses warmed.

Mi-chien-tao-fang 蜜煎導方
(Mel Decoction Formula)

7 *ho*	Mel (Honey)

Put the mel into a bronze container and decoct it over a low flame until it becomes a thick liquid. Stir often to prevent scorching. To make pills (suppositories), knead and form into finger size pellets two inches in length with a sharp head. This should be done quickly while the substance is hot as it becomes hard when cold. Insert the suppositories thus formed into the anus manually. Keep compressing the anus with the hand until an urgent defection sensation ensues. In clinical experiments this formula has been shown to be very effective for hard stools.

Another useful therapy for constipation consists of mixing pig's gall (bile) with vinegar and injecting the combination into the rectum. In one meal's time, the accumulated undigested food and a noxious substance will be discharged.

Yin-chen-hao-tang 茵陳蒿湯
(Capillaris Combination)

6 *liang*	Capillaris
14	Gardenia
3 *liang*	Rhubarb with outer bark removed

Place the capillaris in 1 *tou* 2 *sheng* of water and boil until 6 *sheng* remain. Then add the two remaining herbs and boil down to a volume of 3 *sheng*. Strain and take the prescription in three doses. Diuresis will be induced.

Wu-chu-yu-tang 吳茱萸湯
(Evodia Combination)

1 *sheng*	Evodia, washed
3 *liang*	Ginseng
6 *liang*	Ginger, cut
12	Jujube, shredded

Put the above herbs into 7 *sheng* of water and boil the mixture until only 2 *sheng* remain. Remove the residue and take 7 *ho* of the warmed formula three times daily.

Chih-tzu-po-pi-tang 梔子蘗皮湯
(Gardenia and Phellodendron Combination)

15	Gardenia, cut up (big and fleshy ones preferred)
1 *liang*	Licorice, seared
2 *liang*	Phellodendron

Place the three herbs in 4 *sheng* of water and reduce the amount to 1½ *sheng* by boiling. Strain and take the combination while warm.

Ma-huang-lien-chiao-chih-hsiao-tou-tang

麻黃連翹赤小豆湯

(Ma-huang, Forsythia, and Phaseolus Combination)

2 *liang*	*Ma-huang* with nodes removed
2 *liang*	Forsythia
40	Apricot Seeds with outer skin and apexes removed
1 *sheng*	Phaseolus
12	Jujube, shredded
1 *sheng*	Morus, cut
2 *liang*	Ginger, cut
2 *liang*	Licorice, seared

Place the *ma-huang* in 1 *tou* of clear rain water and boil. Skim off the white froth before adding the remaining herbs. Boil the mixture down to a volume of 3 *sheng*. Strain and take the combination in three separate doses warmed.

Kuei-chih-chia-shao-yao-tang 桂枝加芍藥湯
(Cinnamon and Paeonia Combination)

3 *liang*	Cinnamon with outer bark removed
6 *liang*	Paeonia
3 *liang*	Licorice, seared
12	Jujube, shredded
3 *liang*	Ginger cut

Put the above herbs in 7 *sheng* of water and boil until 3 *sheng*

197

remain. Remove the residue and take the prescription in three separate doses warmed.

Kuei-chih-chia-ta-huang-tang 桂枝加大黃湯
(Cinnamon and Rhubarb Combination)

3 *liang*	Cinnamon with outer bark removed
2 *liang*	Rhubarb
6 *liang*	Paeonia,
3 *liang*	Ginger, cut
2 *liang*	Licorice, seared
12	Jujube, shredded

Place the six herbs in 7 *sheng* of water and reduce the mixture to 3 *sheng* by boiling. Remove the residue and take 1 *sheng* of the formula three times daily warmed.

Ma-huang-hsi-hsin-fu-tzu-tang 麻黃細辛附子湯
(Ma-huang, Asarum, and Aconite Combination)

2 *liang*	*Ma-huang* with nodes removed
2 *liang*	Asarum
1	Aconite, baked with outer bark removed, and cut into eight pieces

Put the *ma-huang* in 1 *tou* of water and boil the contents down to 8 *sheng*. Skim off the white foam and then add the remaining herbs. Boil again until 3 *sheng* remain. Strain and take 1 *sheng* of the combination while warm.

Ma-huang-fu-tzu-kan-tsao-tang 麻黃附子甘草湯
(Ma-huang, Aconite, and Licorice Combination)

2 *liang*	*Ma-huang* with nodes removed
2 *liang*	Licorice, seared
1	Aconite, baked with outer bark removed and cut into eight pieces

198

Place the *ma-huang* in 7 *sheng* of water and boil for a short time. Skim off the white froth and then add the other herbs. Boil the mixture down to 3 *sheng*. Remove the residue and take 1 *sheng* of the prescription while warm.

Huang-lien-ah-chiao-tang 黃連阿膠湯
(Coptis and Gelatin Combination)

4 *liang*	Coptis
2 *liang*	Scute
2 *liang*	Paeonia
2	Egg yolk
3 *liang*	Gelatin

Put the first three herbs in 6 *sheng* of water and boil the contents until only 2 *sheng* remain. Remove the sediment and add the gelatin. Boil again until the latter is well dissolved and then cool. Place the egg yolk into the mixture and blend well. Take 7 *ho* of the formula three times daily warmed.

Fu-tzu-tang 附子湯
(Aconite Combination)

2	Aconite, baked with outer bark removed, and cut into eight pieces
3 *liang*	Hoelen
2 *liang*	Ginseng
4 *liang*	Atractylodes
3 *liang*	Paeonia

Place the above herbs in 8 *sheng* of water and reduce the volume to 3 *sheng* by boiling. Strain and take 1 *sheng* of the combination three times daily warmed.

199

Tao-hua-tang 桃花湯
(Kaolin and Oryza Combination)

1 *chin*   Kaolin, one half being used as presented, the other
           half pulverized and sifted
1 *liang*   Ginger
1 *sheng* Oryza

Put the latter two herbs and the unpulverized half of the first in 7 *sheng* of water and boil until the oryza is well cooked. Remove the residue and add 2 grams of the kaolin powder. Take the prescription three times daily.

Chu-fu-tang 豬膚湯
(Pig's Hide Combination)

1 *chin*   pig's hide

Place the hide in 1 *tou* of water and boil down until 5 *sheng* remains. Remove sediment and add 1 *sheng* of refined mel and 5 *ho* of rice powder. Boil until there is a fragrant odor and the mixture is well blended. Divide the formula into six doses and take warmed.

Kan-tsao-tang 甘草湯
(Licorice Combination)

2 *liang*   Licorice

Place the licorice in 3 *sheng* of water. Reduce the contents to 1½ *sheng* by boiling. Strain and take 7 *ho* of the combination twice daily warmed.

Chieh-keng-tang 桔梗湯
(Platycodon Combination)

1 *liang*   Platycodon

200

2 *liang*   Licorice

Place the herbs in 3 *sheng* of water. Boil the mixture down until only 1 *sheng* remains. Remove the residue and take the prescription in two separate doses while it is warm.

Pan-hsia-ku-chiu-tang 半夏苦酒湯
(Pinellia and Vinegar Combination)

14	Pinellia, washed and cut into pieces the size of date kernels
1	egg white mixed with top quality vinegar and placed in the egg shell

Put the pinellia in the vinegar-egg white mixture in the egg shell. Set the latter on the ring opening of an ancient knife coin and heat until the mixture boils for awhile. Remove the sediment and sip the formula slowly by taking a small quantity in the mouth each time and swallowing it. If the disease (laryngeal tuberculosis) is not improved, prepare and take an additional three doses.

Pan-hsia-san-chi-tang 半夏散及湯
(Pinellia Formula and Combination)

Pinellia, washed
Cinnamon with outer bark removed
Licorice, seared

Pound equal portions of the three herbs, and then sift them separately before combining them. Take 2 grams of the powder with rice congee three times daily. If the patient is unable to take the powder in this manner, put 4 grams of it in 1 *sheng* of boiling water. Bring to a boil again and cook for a short time, cool, then sip the combination.

Pai-tung-tang 白通湯
(Allium, Ginger, and Aconite Combination)

4	Allium
1 *liang*	Ginger
1	Aconite, raw with outer bark removed and cut into eight pieces

Place the above herbs in 3 *sheng* of water. Reduce the volume to 1 *sheng* by boiling. Strain and divide and prescription into two doses and take warmed.

Pai-tung-chia-chu-tan-chih-tang 白通加豬膽汁湯
(A. G. A. and Pig's Bile Combination)

4	Allium
1 *liang*	Ginger
1	Aconite, raw with outer bark removed and cut into eight pieces
5 *ho*	Human urine
1 *ho*	pig's bile

Place the first three herbs in 3 *sheng* of water and boil down until only 1 *sheng* remains. Strain. Add the other herbs and blend well. Take the combination in two doses warmed.

Hsuan-wu-tang 玄武湯
(Vitality Combination)

3 *liang*	Hoelen
3 *liang*	Paeonia
2 *liang*	Atractylodes
3 *liang*	Ginger, cut
1	Aconite, baked to remove outer bark and cut into eight pieces

Put the five herbs in 8 *sheng* of water. Reduce the volume to 3 *sheng* by boiling and remove the residue. Take 7 *ho* of the prescription warmed three times daily.

Tung-mo-szu-ni-tang 通脈四逆湯
(Aconite, Ginger, and Licorice Pulse Combination)

    2 *liang*   Licorice, seared
    1   Aconite (large size), raw with outer bark removed
               and cut into eight pieces
    3 *liang*   Ginger
               (4 *liang* may be used for the strong constitution)

Place the above three herbs in 3 *sheng* of water and boil until only 1 *sheng* and 2 *ho* remain. Remove the sediment and take the formula warmed in two doses.

Szu-ni-san 四逆散
(Bupleurum and Chih-shih Formula)

               Licorice, seared
               Chih-shih, soaked, cut and seared
               Bupleurum
               Paeonia

Pound to a powder equal portions of the four herbs and sift them separately. Take 2 grams of the powder with rice congee three times daily.

Chu-ling-tang 豬苓湯
(Polyporus Combination)

    1 *liang*   Polyporus with outer bark removed
    1 *liang*   Hoelen
    1 *liang*   Alisma
    1 *liang*   Gelatin

Place the first three herbs in 4 *sheng* of water and decrease the amount to 2 *sheng* by boiling. Strain and add the gelatin. Boil until the latter is well dissolved. Take 7 *ho* of the combination warmed three times daily.

Wu-mei-yuan 烏梅圓
(Mume Formula)

300	Mume
6 *liang*	Asarum
10 *liang*	Ginger
16 *liang*	Coptis
4 *liang*	*Tang-kuei*
6 *liang*	Aconite, baked with outer bark removed
4 *liang*	Zanthoxylum, baked
6 *liang*	Cinnamon with outer bark removed
6 *liang*	Ginseng
6 *liang*	Phellodendron

Pound and sift each of the ten herbs separately into powders and then mix together and prepare as follows: Soak the mume overnight in vinegar, remove the kernel, and then steam it with 3 *sheng* of rice is well cooked. Pound the rice together with the mume into a slush and then mix the herb powders in well. Put the formula in a mortar, pour in mel, and pound for 2,000 strokes. Form into pills the size of a dryancra seed. Take ten pills before meals three times daily, gradually increasing the dosage to twenty. Raw, cold food, fats, and odorous dishes are contraindicated during treatment.

Tang-kuei-szu-ni-tang 當歸四逆湯
(Tang-kuei and Jujube Combination)

3 *liang*	*Tang-kuei*
3 *liang*	Cinnamon with outer bark removed
3 *liang*	Paeonia
3 *liang*	Asarum
2 *liang*	Licorice, seared
2 *liang*	Akebia
25	Jujube, shredded

Place the above herbs in 8 *sheng* of water. Reduce the volume to 3 *sheng* by boiling and strain. Take 1 *sheng* of the combination warmed three times daily.

Tang-kuei-szu-ni-chia-wu-chu-yu-sheng-chiang-tang

當歸四逆加吳茱萸生薑湯

(Tang-kuei, Evodia, and Ginger Combination)

3 *liang*	Tang-kuei
3 *liang*	Paeonia
2 *liang*	Licorice, seared
2 *liang*	Akebia
3 *liang*	Cinnamon with outer bark removed
3 *liang*	Asarum
½ *chin*	Ginger, cut
2 *liang*	Evodia
25	Jujube, shredded

Put the above herbs in 6 *sheng* of water and 6 *sheng* of wine. Boil the mixture until the contents is reduced to 5 *sheng*. Remove the residue and take the prescription in five doses warmed.

Kan-chiang-huang-chin-huang-lien-jen-sheng-tang

乾薑黃芩黃連人參湯

(Ginger and S. C. G. Combination)

3 *liang*	Ginger
3 *liang*	Scute
3 *liang*	Coptis
3 *liang*	Ginseng

Place the above herbs in 6 *sheng* of water and boil the contents until only 2 *sheng* remain. Remove the sediment and take the formula in two separate doses warmed.

Pai-tou-weng-tang 白頭翁湯
(Anemone Combination)

2 *liang*   Anemone
3 *liang*   Phellodendron
3 *liang*   Coptis
3 *liang*   Fraxinus

Place the above herbs in 7 *sheng* of water and boil down to 2 *sheng*. Remove the residue and bake 1 *sheng* warmed. If recovery is not achieved, take one more *sheng*.

Szu-ni-chia-jen-sheng-tang 四逆加人參湯
(Ginseng, Aconite, and Licorice Combination)

2 *liang*   Licorice, seared
1   Aconite, raw with outer bark removed, and cut into eight pieces
1½ *liang* Ginger
1 *liang*   Ginseng

Put the four herbs in 3 *sheng* of water and boil down until 1 *sheng* 2 *ho* remain. Strain and take the combination in two equal doses warmed.

Li-chung-wan 理中丸
(Ginseng and Ginger Formula)

3 *liang*   Ginseng
3 *liang*   Ginger
3 *liang*   Licorice, seared
3 *liang*   Atractylodes

Pound the four herbs into a powder and sift. Mix them with mel to form yolk size pills. Grind one pill into pieces and put into several *ho* of boiling water. Take the formula while warm. If there is no increase of heat in the abdomen, increase the dosage to 3 or 4 pills at one time but with the same amount of boiling water. If the combination is to be taken in decoction form, it is prepared as follows: cut the herbs into pieces and put them in 8 *sheng* of water; boil down to a volume of 3 *sheng;* strain and take 1 *sheng* of the prescription three times daily warmed.

Tung-mo-Szu-ni-chia-chu-tan-chih-tang

通脉四逆加豬膽汁湯

(L. A. Ginger and Pig's Bile Combination)

3 *liang*	Licorice, seared
3 *liang*	Ginger
	(or 4 *liang* in strong constitution cases)
1	Aconite, raw with outer bark removed and cut into 8 pieces
½ *ho*	pig's bile

Boil the first 3 herbs with 3 *sheng* of water until 1 *sheng* remains. Remove the residue and stir in the bile. Take the combination in two separate doses warmed.

Chih-shih-chih-tzu-tang 枳實梔子湯
(Chih-shih and Gardenia Combination)

3	*Chih-shih,* seared
14	Gardenia, shredded
1 *sheng*	Soja, wrapped in silk cloth

Boil 7 *sheng* of clear rice soup down to a volume of 4 *sheng*. Add the first two herbs and further boil until the amount is 2 *sheng*. Then put in the soja and reboil 5 or 6 times. Strain and take the formula in two separate doses warmed.

Mu-li-tse-hsieh-san 牡蠣澤瀉散
(Oyster Shell and Alisma Formula)

Oyster shell, simmered

Alisma

Dichroa, washed to remove its offensive odor

Lepidium, simmered
Phytolacca, simmered
Sargassum, washed to remove saltiness
Trichosanthes root

Pound and sift equal portions of each of the above herbs separately into powder. Place in a mortar and blend thoroughly. Take 2 grams of the powder with rice soup three times daily. In the event of diuresis, discontinue taking.

Chu-yeh-shih-kao-tang 竹葉石膏湯
(Bamboo Leaves and Gypsum Combination)

2 handfuls	Bamboo leaves
1 *chin*	Gypsum
½ *sheng*	Pinellia, washed
1 *sheng*	Ophiopogon, decored
2 *liang*	Ginseng
2 *liang*	Licorice, seared
½ *sheng*	Oryza

Place the first six herbs in 1 *tou* of water. Reduce the volume to 6 *sheng* by boiling. Remove the sediment and then add the oryza. Boil again until the latter is well cooked. Strain. Take 1 *sheng* of the prescription three times daily warmed.

The Units of Measurement

The dosages recorded in the *Shang han lun* have been a matter of controversy since ancient times. Keisetsu favors the opinions of Koshima Gako, Kitamura Kousou, Yamada Tsintei et al. who believe in the research and verification that holds that the measurements and weights can be converted to modern day equivalents. Koshima Gako says, "In ancient times, ten *shus* (黍) equalled one *lei* (絫); ten *leis* (絫) equalled one *chu* (銖); and proportionately the higher units were *liang* (兩) and *chin* (斤) These are also the currently used weight units. The field of medicine uses one-tenth of these units for measurement, this system being referred to as *Shen Nung's* weights.

When Japanese grown millet is used to check the actual weights (the bigger grains being selected for the weighing), then one ancient *chin* (斤) equals five *chiens* (錢), five *fens* (分), six *lis* (釐), and eight *haos* (毫) in current weights. Also, according to current weights, one *chin* (斤) equals sixteen *liangs* (兩) and one *liangs* (兩) equals twenty-four *chus* (銖). By further calculation, one *chu* (銖) equals one *li* (釐), four *haos* (毫), and five *szu* (絲); and one *liang* (兩) equals three *fens* (分), four *lis* (釐) and eight *haos* (毫).

Tao Yin-chu said in his *Pen ts'ao hsu li* (General Notes for the Preface of the *Pen ts'ao*): "In ancient times the steelyard was graduated into *chu* (銖) and *liang* (兩) without the finer gradation of *fen* (分). Presently, the *shus* (黍) equal one *chu* (銖); eight *chus* (銖) equal one *fen* (分); four *fens* (分) equal one *liang* (兩); and sixteen *liang* (兩) equal one *chin* (斤)."

In accordance with the above relationships, the following tables of comparison (see tables 2-5) can be made:

Table 2 The Unit of *Chu* (銖)

| Han Dynasty—China | Tokugawa Era—Japan | | | | | Present Day |
chu (銖)	chien (錢)	fen (分)	li (釐)	hao (毫)	szu (絲)	grams
1			1	4	5	ca. 0.05
2			2	9		0.10
3			4	3	5	0.16
4			5	8		0.20
5			7	2	5	0.27
6			8	7		0.30
7		1		1	5	0.37
8		1	1	6		0.40
9		1	3		5	0.48
10		1	4		5	0.50

Table 3 The Unit of *Liang* (兩)

| Han Dynasty—China | Tokugawa Era—Japan | | | | | Present Day |
liang	chien	fen	li	hao	szu	grams
1		3	4	8		1.30
2		6	9	6		2.70
3	1		4	4		3.90
3	1	3	9	2		5.20
5	1	7	8			6.60
6	2	8	8			7.80
7	2	4	3	6		9.00
8	2	7	8	4		10.40
9	3	1	3	2		11.70
10	3	4	8			13.00

Table 4
The Unit of *Chin* (斤)

Han Dynasty—China	Tokugawa Era—Japan					Present Day
chin	*chien*	*fen*	*li*	*hao*	*szu*	grams
1	5	5	6	8		20.80
2	11	1	3	6		41.70

Table 5
The Unit of *Fen* (分)

Han Dynasty—China	Tokugawa Era—Japan					Present Day
fen	*chien*	*fen*	*li*	*hao*	*szu*	grams
1			8	7		ca. 0.3
2		1	7	4		0.6
3		2	6	1		1.0
4		3	4	8		1.3
5		4	3	5		1.6
6		5	2	2		2.0
7		6		9		2.3
8		6	9	6		2.6
9		7	8	3		2.9
10		8	7			3.2

211

Table 6
Weights and Measures Used in Present Day Chinese
Market System

1 *chin* (斤) = 16 *liang* (兩) = 500.0000 grams
1 *liang* (兩) = 10 *chien* (錢) = 31.2500 grams
1 *chien* (錢) = 10 *fen* (分) = 3.1250 grams
1 *fen* (分) = 10 *li* (釐) = 0.3125 grams
1 *li* (釐) = 0.0313 grams
1 *tou* (斗) = 10 *sheng* (升) = 10.0000 liters (ten)
1 *sheng* (升) = 10 *ho* (合) = 1.0000 liter (one)
1 *ho* (合) = 0.1000 liter
1 *chang* (丈) = 10 *ch'ih* (尺) = about 3.333 meters
1 *ch'ih* (尺) = 10 *ts'un* (寸) = about 0.3333 meter
1 *ts'un* (寸) = 10 *fen* (分) = about 0.0333 centimeters
1 *fen* (分) = about 0.0033 centimeters

The Unit of *Fen* (分)

There are two meanings to the character *fen* (分) as used in the medical field: one is the division or separation of things or medicines into smaller portions, having nothing to do with weighing; the other is the weighing unit in relation to one *fen* (分) being equal to six *chus* (銖). The relationships of the *fen* (分) are shown in the following table (see Table 5).

The Measuring Vessel — *Yao sheng* (藥升)

Tao Yin-chu said, "*Yao sheng*, the measuring vessel for drugs, has the dimensions of one *tsun* (寸, about one inch) for each side of the upper square, eight *fens* (about eight-tenths of an inch) for each side of the lower square and a height of six *fens*. Owing to differences in density of drugs, it is rather difficult to convert this volume into the corresponding weights in *chin* (斤) and *liang* (兩).

Koshima Gako said, "After investigating Chang Chung-ching's formulas, I found that the medicines such as mirabilitum, ophiopogon, pinellia, red mung bean, the raw white bark of *tzu,* the

212

white cortex of sweet plum root, evodia, wheat, apricot, linum kernel, gadfly, scarab larva, cockroach, schizandra fruit, reed stem, coix, gourd melon seed, zizyphus, and white protion of bamboo stem were given in dosages measured by *yao Sheng*. While maltose jelly, raw rehmannia, horse urine, human milk, decoction of water from rice washing and perilla, gourd melon juice, human feces juice, earth slurry, hard sugar, salt, honey, clear wine, bitter wine, and white wine were administered in dosages of the same units as are used presently, instead of in *yao sheng* units. Also the measurement of so many *hos* of unglutinous rice is the same unit as the one presently used.

Present Day Equivalents of Units Used in the *Shang han lun*

1 *tou* (斗)	slightly more than 10 *sheng* ca. 2000 ml. (升) and 1 *ho* (合)
1 *sheng* (升)	slightly more than 10 *sheng* 200 (升) and 1 *shao* (勺)
1 *ho* (合)	slightly more than 10 *shao* (勺) 20
1 large *chang* (盞)	about 1 *sheng* (升)
1 average *chang* (盞)	about 5 *ho* (合)
1 small *chang* (盞)	about 3 *ho* (合)

A one-inch square spoon is a square medicinal spoon having the dimensions of one inch in length, breadth, and height. It is used to scoop and measure as much a quantity of medicinal powder as will not brim over the spoon. However, as drugs differ in density, the measured drugs may weigh from 1.5 grams in some cases to about 2.5 in others. Now it is used to measure an equivalent of 2.0 grams.

A one-stone spatula holds about one-tenth the volume of the one-inch square spoon.

A one-coin spoon is named for the five *chu* coin used in the Han dynasty. It holds as much medicinal powder as the coin can retain without brimming over. The weight of medicines so measured is inaccurate due to differences in density. It is now used to measure amounts equivalent to 1.0 grams.

213

Sterculia-seed size refers to the quanity of medicinal powder contained in a one-inch square spoon. The powder is then mixed with honey and made into pills of the size of a sterculia seed. Ten pills can be produced from the above amount with each pill weighing about 0.2 grams.

Bullet size refers to a pill weighing 2.0 grams, ten times larger than sterculia-seed size.

Egg yolk size is the same size as bullet size, 2.0 grams.

Croton-seed size is the size of a croton seed which varies; the weight of the seed decreases when stored due to the natural loss of liquid. According to *Notes for the Preface fo Pen ts'ao*, sixteen seeds whose germs and coarse skins have been removed have a total weight of 1 *fen*. Today if we take sixteen seeds similarly treated and weigh them, they will weigh just a little over eight *fens* or about three grams.

Aconite size, according to *Notes for the Preface of Pen ts'ao*, is the size of one peeled aconite, the equivalent of half a *liang* or about 0.5 grams. However, since the size of aconite varies from one to another, this size is also indefinite.

Bitter-orange size, according to *Notes for the Preface of Pen ts'ao*, is equal to two bitter oranges or one *fen* or about three grams. Kitamura Kousou, however, said two pieces equalled five *fens*. The problem lies in that we are not sure of whether the bitter orange used in the time of the writing of the *Shang han lun* is the same as the present day bitter orange. (Since this occurs not only with this drug, but with all others, we must base our weighing units of drugs on the same basis as that adopted for the drugs in the Han dynasty, in order to end the disagreement about drug dosages. However, it is still necessary to know the approximate weight of each unit used.

Jujube size, according to *Notes for the Preface of Pen ts'ao*, indicates that three jujubes are approximately one gram.

Pinellia size says in *Notes for the Preface of Pen ts'ao* is one *sheng* of pinellia weights about five grams or five *liangs*.

Szechuan pepper size in *The Notes* is one *sheng* of this fruit which weighs three *liangs* or three grams.

Evodia size in *The Notes* is one *sheng* of evodia which weighs five *liangs* or about five grams.

Gypsum of an egg's size was taken by Taki Genken to mean three *chiens* or about nine grams.

Ten apricot seeds refers to ten peeled seeds weighing eight *fens* or about three grams.

Ophiopogon size resembles pinellia in that one *sheng* of this drug weighs five *liangs* or about five grams.

One trichosanthes fruit is equivalent to three *fens* or one gram.

One gardenia fruit is equal to three *fens* or about one gram.

One handful of bamboo leaves in *The Notes* is equal to two *liangs* or about two grams.

Glossary

Anemophobia (惡風). Also translated as "mild chills" in this work. This term is a subjective symptom characterized by a morbid dread of drafts or winds, a condition known as hypersensitivity in modern medicine. It is taken into consideration—together with other symptoms such as severe chills, fever, perspiration, and headache—in the diagnosis and determination of a confirmation in Chinese medicine. It represents a mild condition of a cold and is believed to have been contracted as a result of exposure to the wind while sweating. The Chinese term " 微惡寒 " has been translated as "slight chills" or "mild chills," which is a milder condition of severe chills. No matter whether mild chills or severe chills, it represents a shivering or chilly sensation that seems to have been generated from the depths of the body and is always a prelude to an ensuing fever. This condition is the body's self-protective reaction because in the process of a chill, the cells are mobilized, heat is generated, and circulation is accelerated, making more energy available for driving out the ailing toxins. It is then evident that anemophobia and mild chills are two different symptoms,

216

the former being superficial and a hypersensitivity and the latter, internal and a self-protective reaction; otherwise the author would not have used two different terms.

Ch'i (氣). One of the three humors—*ch'i*, blood, and water. Variously translated as vigor, energy, or vitality. In theory it is an air-like, ephemeral substance that circulates throughout the body much like blood does. It may be equated somewhat with nerves in its physical properties and qualities, but it also has a philosophical connotation.

Ching-lo (經絡). The meridians or conduits. Those going in the longitudinal direction are known as *ching;* whereas those going transversely and interconnecting the *ching* meridians are named *lo*.

Chung feng (中風). A mild feverish condition of greater yang disease characterized by the symptoms indicated in Article 2, Part II.

Confirmation (證). A comprehensive identification, hence a holistic treatment of a pathic condition based on the subjective and objective symptoms in an individual (not necessarily a patient). The confirmation changes as the symptoms change thus the treatment changes too.

Five Elements (五行). Wood, water, fire, earth, and metal. In Chinese philosophy:
water produces wood but destroys fire
fire produces earth but destroys metal
metal produces water but destroys wood
wood produces fire but destroys earth
earth produces metal but destroys water

Five Viscera or Five Solid Organs (五臟). The five viscera are the heart, liver, kidney, spleen, and lungs. They either govern or are governed by the five elements.

Viscera	Element
heart	fire
liver	wood
spleen	earth
lungs	metal
kidneys	water

Inside (裡). Internal parts of the body; or internal symptoms or confirmations; the opposite of outside or external. A disease that is inside has affected the viscera and is more

217

serious than an outside disease.

Outside or Surface (表). External parts of the body; the visible surface of the body. An outside or surface disease is less serious than an inside disease.

Purgation (下). The act of causing bowel movement. An important type of treatment in Chinese medicine.

***Shang han* (傷寒).** A condition of a cold characterized by the symptoms indicated in Article 3, Part II.

Stagnancy (停滯). The occlusion or stoppage of the circulation of blood, water, or *ch'i*.

Tide fever (潮熱). A fever that comes and goes, ebbs and wanes like the tide.

Volumes (卷). Ancient Chinese literature was hand scripted on scrolls or rolls. Each roll is considered to be a book or volume, even though the length of a chapter only. For this reason, to the Western reader each written work sounds like it is the length of a set of encyclopedias whereas in truth it is the length of a normal book, the volume equating to chapters.

Yang (陽). The active, positive, masculine force or principle in the universe; source of light and heat.

Yin (陰). The passive, negative, feminine force or principle in the universe.

Bibliography

Chinese Sources

Chang Hsi-chun. *Shang han lun chiang i* (Lectures on the *Shang han lun*).

傷寒論講義, 1978. A modern work.

Chen Chi-wen. *Shang han lun hsin shih* (A New Explanation of the *Shang han lun*).

傷寒論新釋, 1952. A contemporary work.

Shen Chun-fa. *Shang han lun hsin chieh* (A New Interpretation of the *Shang han lun*).

傷寒論新解, 1977. Another modern work.

Chen Chun-jen. *Chung kuo yao hsuen ta t'su tien* (Chinese Herbal Dictionary).

中國藥學大辭典, 1979. An extensive lexicon that took four years to compile. Entries include original name, nomenclature, formula names, ancient names, scientific names, origin, habitat, morphology, variety, processing method, uses, properties, taste, effects, actions, chief indications, history, foreign theories, compatibilities and incompatibilities, and dosages.

Chen Lao-twei. *Shang han lun shih i* (The Meaning of *Shang han lun*).

傷寒論實義 , 1976. A contemporary explanation.

Chu Tao-hsing. *Shang han kuan chu chih* (A String of Beads on the *Shang han lun*).

傷寒貫珠子 Compiled between 1788-1820. A popular work on the subject; collated by the author and annotated by Yu Tsai-ching.

Fang Yuo-chih; Yu Chan; Ko Chin. *Shang han lun san chung* (Three Works on the *Shang han lun*).

傷寒論三種, 1977. An edition of three separate works, one of which was written in the Ming dynasty and the other two in the Ching dynasty respectively. Each work gives creative opinions that sharply rebuke the errors of former scholars.

Hsieh Kuan. *Chung kuo i hsueh ta ts'u tien* (Chinese Medical Dictionary).

中國醫學大辭典, 1921. The author spent six years on this work, referring to over two thousand works in Chinese, Japanese, and Korean. Over seven thousand entries are listed.

Hsu Hong-yen. *Chang yung chung yao chih yen chiu* (A Study of Chinese Herbal Medicine).

常用中藥之研究, 1972. A description of many herbs and their origins. Includes the identification of several herbs' origins that up until now have been questionable.

Hsu Hong-yen. *Chung yao cheng fen tsui chin yen chiu.* (Recent Advances in the Study of Chinese Herbal Medicine) 中藥成分最近研究 . Taipei: *Kuo li chung kuo i hsueh yen chiu suo*, 1968.

Hsu Hong-yen. *Chung yao chih p'ao-chih* (Methods of Processing Chinese Herbal Drugs).

中藥之炮炙 , 1979. A summary of the methods used to process Chinese herbal drugs (of herbal, animal, or mineral origin). The origin and international scientific name for each drug are given.

Hsu Hong-yen. *K'uang wu hsing chung yao yen chiu* (A Study of Chinese Mineral Drugs) 鑛物性中藥研究 . Taipei: *Kuo li chung kuo i yao yen chiu suo*, 1975. A description of drugs of mineral origin.

Hsu Hong-yen. *Tung-wu hsing chung yao chih yen chiu* (A

220

Study of Chinese Animal Drugs) 動物性中藥之研究 . Taipei: *Kuo li chung kuo i yao yen chiu suo*, 1977. A description of commonly and rarely used drugs of animal origin, along with their history of use, morphological description, habitats, pharmacological actions, and clinical tests.

Hsu Su-wei and Ho Lien-chen. *Tseng ting shang han pai chen ko chu* (A Revised and Expanded Lyrical Annotation on One Hundred Confirmations of the *Shang han lun*). 增訂傷寒百證歌註, 1928. A reference by Hsu Su-wei of the Sung dynasty that was revised by Ho Lien-chen in 1928.

I Lin et al. *Huang ti nei ching su wen* (The Yellow Emperor's Classic of Internal Medicine). 黃帝內經素問, 1117. The supreme authority of Chinese medicine supposedly written by the founder of China. This edition was collated during the Sung dynasty. Nearly all terms and theories concerning internal medicine come from this guide.

I tsung chin chien (The Golden Mirror of Chinese Medicine). 醫宗金鑑, 1741. A compendium of the essential works of Chinese medicine, including the *Shang han lun*. Compiled by royal physicians under the direction of Wu Chien by order of the Emperor during the Ching dynasty.

Ko Chin. *Shan han lai su chih* (The Elucidation of the *Shang han lun*). 傷寒來蘇集 Compiled between 1736-1799. Illuminating articles on Chinese medical theory.

Li Shih-chen. *Tu chieh pen tsao kang mu* (Materia Medica). 圖解本草綱目, 1578. A catalog of 1,892 herbs and 8,160 prescriptions written by a great herbalist of China during the Ming dynasty. The author spent twenty years locating and identifying the many herbs and studied most of the available literature before writing this book.

Oda Kenzo. *Shang han lun keng kai* (An Outline of the *Shang han lun*). 傷寒論梗蓋, 1976. A guide to only the most basic concepts of the *Shang han lun*.

Otsuka Keisetsu. *Shang han lun chieh-shuo* (A Study of the *Shang han lun*).

傷寒論解說, 1966. The original on which this translation is based. Otsuka is one of the foremost authorities on Chinese medicine in Japan. The Chinese edition of the Japanese original was primarily used for our work.

Pao Shih-sheng. *Shang han lun chiang i* (Lectures on the *Shang han lun*).
傷寒論講義, 1975. A contemporary work written in the form of questions and answers.

Shen Nung. *Shen nung pen tsao ching* (Shen Nung's Herbal).
神農本草經, 1875-1908. A nineteenth century edition of the legendary Shen Nung's classic. Believed to be the oldest herbal. Records 360 herbs ranked into three categories: superior, common, inferior. Each category contains 120 herbs. Lists each herb's properties and taste.

Tan Tzu-chung. *Shang han lun ping chu* (A Commentary on the *Shang han lun*).
傷寒論評註, 1970. An explanation by a contemporary Chinese herb physician.

Ting Tu-pao. *Shuo wen chieh tzu ku lin* (Instruction on the Etymology of Chinese Characters).
說文解字詁林, 1930. Sixteen books which are the basic grammar for study of Chinese characters.

Tsiang Tso-ching. *Shang han lun ching chieh tu pen* (A Condensed, Concise Text of the *Shang han lun*).
傷寒論精解圖本, 1968. An interpretation by a contemporary Chinese herbal physician who has incorporated his clinical experiments in the work.

Tu Chung-min. *Chung i yao hsueh ping lun* (A Commentary on Chinese Herbal Medicine).
中醫藥學評論, 1971. A historic review of Chinese herbal medicine from ancient times to the present by the superintendent of the Medical College, National Taiwan University. Accurate, concise, and creative.

Wang Ken-tang. *I tung chen mo chuan shu* (Orthodox Chinese Medicine).
醫通診脈纂疏 Compiled between 1573-1620. An encyclopedic set that includes many important works from physicians and gives a large portion of space to the *Shang han lun*.

Wu Kuo-ting. *Shang han lun ch'uan shih* (An Annotation

on the *Shang han lun*).

傷寒論詮釋 , 1964. Articles commenting on Tanha Genkin's *A Compendium on the Meaning of the Shang han lun* by a professor of Chinese medicine at the China Medical College; Taichung, Taiwan. A primary reference for this translation.

Yeiyo Nishiyam. *Jih hua i hsueh tz'u tien* (Chinese Medical Terminology).

日華醫學辭典 3d ed. 1975.

Yu Ken-chu. *T'ung su shang han lun* (The Popular *Shang han lun*).

通俗傷寒論 , 1878. An easy-to-read interpretation of the *Shang han lun* written in the Ching dynasty.

Yu Wu-yen. *Shang han lun hsin i* (New Meanings of the *Shang han lun*).

傷寒論新義 , 1941. An interpretation of the *Shang han lun* in terms of modern medicine and Chinese medical theories.

English Publications and Sources

Donald's Illustrated Medical Dictionary. 25th ed.: 1974.

Hsu Hong-yen. *Chinese Herbs and Formulas.* Los Angeles: Oriental Healing Arts Institute, 1978. A listing of the most frequently used Chinese herbs, together with formulas in which they are used. Also includes confirmations for the formulas.

Hsu Hong-yen. *How to Treat Yourself with Chinese Herbs.* Los Angeles: Oriental Healing Arts Institute, 1980. An outline of diagnosis, confirmation identification, and treatment of disease according to herbal formulas, some of which come from the *Shang han lun.*

Hsu Hong-yen and Peacher, William. *Chen's History of Chinese Medical Science.* Los Angeles: Oriental Healing Arts Institute, 1977. The biographies of renowned Chinese physicians.

Hsu Hong-yen and Peacher, William. *Chinese Herb Medicine and Therapy.* Los Angeles: Oriental Healing Arts Institute, 1976. An orientation to the basic principles of Chinese medicine and a stepping stone to more extensive study.

Liang Shih-chiu. *A New Practical Chinese-English Dictionary*. Taipei: The Far East Book Co., Ltd., 1973.

Nanzando's Medical Dictionary. 10th ed. 南山堂醫學大辭典 , 1964. A Japanese-English lexicon.

Smith, T. Porter and G. A. Stuart, *Chinese Medicinal Herbs*. San Francisco: Georgetown Press, 1973. Originally published in 1911; an English translation of Li Shih-chen's *Pen ts'ao Kang mu* (Materia Medica).

Stuart, G. A. *A Chinese Materia Medica*. Taipei: Southern Materials Center, 1976. A set of books based on the investigations and research of T. Porter Smith on plant, animal, and mineral drugs found in *Pen ts'ao kang mu*. Lists the scientific name, generic name, Chinese name, part used, constituents, references, descriptions, identification, and processing method for each drug.

Veith, Ilza. *The Yellow Emperor's Classic of Internal Medicine* (*Nei ching*). Berkeley: University of California Press, 1965. An English translation of Chapters 1-34 of the classic with an introductory study.

Webster's New World Dictionary. 2d college ed. Editor in Chief David B. Guralnik. Cleveland: William Collins Publishers, 1978.

Appendixes

Appendix 1

Su Wen

Further information is found in the "Treatise on the Canons and Literature." *Su wen* represents nine rolls of the *Nei ching* (The Yellow Emperor's Classic of Internal Medicine) with an additional nine rolls comprising the *Ling shu* (Mystical Pivot) making a total of eighteen rolls.

Prior to the renewed interest in acupuncture in the United States in 1972, there was only one partial translation of the *Nei ching* written in English. Ilza Veith translated the first thirty-four chapters—the *Su wen* (the first half of the *Nei ching*) — in 1949 which has been widely reprinted since 1966. There is an excellent preface, introduction, and bibliography, as well as three instructive appendices: Chapter 103 of the *Ssu k'u ch'uan shu*; preface of the commentator Wang Ping (A.D. 762); and preface of Kao Pao-heng and Lin I (A.D. 1078).

The final form of the *Nei ching*, which is in two sections, is attributed to Wang Ping (A.D. 762). This text survives to this day. Wang Man, however, feels that the version now commonly used is a rearrangement of an edition by Chang Yin-an and Ma Yuan-tai of the Ming dynasty (1368-1644).

Wang Man in an article in the *Chinese Medical Journal*;

Volume 68, pages 1-33; (1950) comments on his theories as to the date of origin and authorship of the *Nei ching*. As noted here, Chang Chung-ching in his preface gave the first recorded evidence of this treatise when he referred to the *"Su wen* in nine volumes." The second half of the *Nei ching*, the *Ling shu*, was identified as the "Classic of Acupuncture" by Huang Fu-mi in A.D. 265 and as the "Nine Volumes" by Wang Shu-ho in A.D. 370. The *Nei ching* was referred to as the "Nine Ling," and "Acupuncture Classic," in the "Record of Books and Classics" in the *Annals of Sui* (A.D. 622). In 762 Wang Ping called it the *"Ling shu"* which means the "spiritual gate" or "living center" or "mystical pivot."

The *Nei ching* is thought to have been written after the death of Confucius in 479 B.C. and infused with the doctrines of yin and yang, numerology, and the Five Elements in the early Han dynasty (206 B.C. − A.D. 9) as mentioned in the *Record of Arts and Letters* by Pan Ku (A.D. 79). The material on "Vapors" and "Airs" as propounded by Tung Chung-shu in A.D. 150 became incorporated into the thesis in the Chin dynasty (A.D. 268-420).

Veith's *Nei ching* will give the occidental unfamiliar with the Chinese language a general knowledge concerning the practice of medicine in early China. This work covers every branch of medicine and allied subjects: astrology, geography, humanities, hygiene, anatomy, physiology, etiology, symptomatology, pathology, nutrition, diagnosis, prognosis, and prevention and treatment of disease. The *Su wen* covers the natural history of illness, its diagnosis, prognosis, and prevention rendered in the form of a series of questions and answers, and the *Ling shu* deals primarily with treatment, largely acupuncture. Anatomy and physiology are stressed. Unfortunately, there is much overlap and frequent repetition in both sections. The *Su wen* propounds two basic concepts of health and disease.

1. The normal function of the body depends upon an equilibrium of yin and yang, the two vital principles that permeate the whole of nature.
2. Nature and man contain a mixture of five substances— wood, fire, earth, metal, and water—which interact and determine one's state of being.

Further, both of the above basic mechanisms are correlated

with the solid and hollow organs which in turn reflect disease states and disturbances of the physiology as demonstrated by the four cardinal methods of diagnosis: observation, questioning, listening, and palpation of the pulse and abdomen. The importance of the pulse in the diagnosis of the type and location of disease and its prognosis is emphasized in the *Nei ching's Su wen*. Four principal pulses are described: (1) *fu* - superficial; (2) *ch'en* - deep; (3) *ch'ih* - slow; and (4) *shu* - quick. There are three sets of pulses on each hand that are palpated superficially or externally to diagnose the yang organs and deeply or internally to diagnose the yin organs. The one most distal or closest to the wrist is named *tsun* (inch), the next *kuan* (bar), and the most proximal *ch'ih* (cubit). The various factors influencing the pulse are clearly delineated as to the seasons, time of day, wind, and evil or noxious air. The subdivisions of yang -- greater, lesser, and sunlight -- and yin -- greater, lesser, and absolute -- are correlated also with the various subdivisions of the pulse. This important work must have been of tremendous benefit to Chang in his preparation of the *Shang han tsa ping lun*.

Henry C. Lu of the Academy of Oriental Heritage in Vancouver, British Columbia, Canada, translated the first fourteen chapters of the *Ling shu* into English in 1974. He is currently rendering the entire *Nei ching* into this language, including Volume V, the "Difficult Classic". Besides the translation, he interprets assertions made in the *Nei ching*. The book will have twenty-two questions concerning the pulse, seven questions on the meridians, eighteen questions on the viscera and bowels, fourteen questions on diseases, seven questions on acupuncture points, and the remaining thirteen questions on techniques of acupuncture. Each chapter includes the key concepts, the Chinese text, the English translation, the translator's commentary, and illustrations.

Other investigators planning currently to put the *Nei ching* into English include Drs. Frederick F. Kao of New York and Nguyen Van Nighi of Marseilles, France, and another interested group of investigators in Florida. So far as European translators of the *Nei ching* are concerned, Hubotter has made an incomplete transcription into German. A. Chamfrault published *Treatise on Chinese Medicine* in French in 1957 and a second edition in 1964; he co-authored Volume II of the same title with M. Ung

Kang Sam which is a complete translation of the *Nei ching* (*Su wen* and *Ling shu*), including a table of contents containing a brief summary of each chapter.

Appendix 2

Nan ching

This short treatise consists of explanations of annotations on eighty-one difficult passages selected from the *Nei ching*. It has been attributed to Pien ch'iao (Pien Chueh; Chin Yueh-jen ca. 407-310 B.C.). As mentioned above, Lu's is the current translation of this work in English. It is available also in German through the efforts of Hubotter.

Appendix 3

"Yin yang ying hsiang ta lung"
(The Great Treatise of Yin and Yang)
and
A Summary of Ancient References
to
Yin and Yang

In the *Han shu* (History of the Former Han Dynasty) in the section "Treatise on the Canons and Literature" by Pan Ku, there were eighteen books listed as comprising the *Huang ti nei ching*. As has been noted, Chang quoted this work and apparently was the first to call it *Su wen*. Huang-fu Mi (A.D. 215-286), author of the *Chia i ching*, the only ancient Chinese acupuncture book that has survived intact through the generations, affirmed also the existence of eighteen books of the *Nei ching*. We find the name of "*Su wen*" recorded in the *Annals of the Sui Dynasty* (A.D. 589-618), but only eight books were mentioned in the *Record of Books*. Then Wang Ping (ca. A.D. 762) in the reign of Pao Ying of the T'ang dynasty (A.D. 618-907) substituted a missing chapter from an ancient edition. This chapter is felt to represent the same "Great Treatise of Yin and Yang" mentioned here by Chang.

Other works that were available to Chang contained some information on yin and yang. These are listed here. The philosophical use of the terms began in the beginning of the fourth century B.C.

    a. *Kuo yu* (Discussion of the States) ca. fourth or fifth

231

century B.C. An earthquake occurring in 780 B.C. was explained in the following terms: "When the yang is concealed and cannot come forth, and when the yin is repressed and cannot issue forth, then there are earthquakes." (*"Chou yu"*, I, 10)

b. *Tsou yen* (350-270 B.C.), proponent and possible originator of the Five Element theory, did not mention the two fundamental forces nor can anything be found on the subject in surviving fragments of his work.

c. *I ching* (The Book of Changes), Chou dynasty with additions made in the Han dyansty, compiler unknown. In Appendix 5, Chapter 5 (*Hsi Tz'u*, the Great Appendix) from the late Warring State Period (403-221 B.C.), the statement is made, "One yin and one yang – that is the *Tao.*" In later times the theory of yin and yang became associated primarily with the *I ching* where the relationship of yin and yang with numbers and the five elements was stressed. Originally a book of divinination, it was later given cosmological, metaphysical,and ethical interpretations by Confucianists.

d. *Mo tzu* (The Book of the Master Mo, Master Mo Ti, and His Disciples); Chou dynasty, fourth century B.C. There are two references to yin and yang. In Chapter 6, Mo tzu states that every living creature partakes of the nature of heaven and earth and of the harmony of the yin and the yang. In Chapter 27, the virtue of the sage kings was said to have brought yin and yang, the rain and the dew, at timely seasons.

e. *Nan hua chen ching* (The Book of Master Chuang) by Chang tzu, Chou dynasty ca. 290 B.C. The dual phenomenon of yin and yang is mentioned frequently, occurring at least in twenty different passages of the text.

f. *Tao te ching* (Canon of the Virtue of the Tao); Chou dynasty before 300 B.C. This book has been attributed to Li Erh (Lao Tzu). Yin and yang are mentioned in Chapter 42 where it states that living creatures are surrounded by yin and envelop yang, and that harmony of their life processes depends upon harmony of these two *ch'i*.

g. *Shu ching* (Historical Classic – Book of Documents). The twenty-nine *Chin wen* chapters are mainly of the Chou dynasty with a few sections possibly dating from the Shang period. Thirteen of the chapters are felt to date to the tenth century B.C.; ten to the eighth century B.C.; and six not before the fifth century B.C. Some scholars accept only sixteen or seventeen as pre-Confucian. The twenty-one *Ku wen* chapters with fragments of genuine antiquity supposedly infused were regarded as a forgery by Mei Tse, ca. A.D. 320. This book was translated by W. H. Medhurst in 1846, J. Legge in 1865, and B. Karlgren in 1950.

h. *Tso chuan*; Master Tso Ch'iu-ming's commentary on the *Chuen Chiu* (Spring and Autumn Annals); Chou dynasty, compiled between 430 and 250 B.C. Additions and changes were made by Confucian scholars of the sections on the Chin and Han periods, especially by Liu Hsin. This book covers the period of 722-453 B.C. and is the greatest of the three commentaries on the *Chuen Chiu*. The others are *Kung yang chuan* and *Kuliang chuan*, but they differ from the above which was written originally as a book of history; translated by J. Legge in 1872 and F. S. Couvreur in 1951.

i. *Hsun ching*, (The Book of Master Hsun) by Hsun Tzu, Chou dynasty ca. 240 B.C., translated by H. H. Dubs, 1927.

j. *Hsiao tai li chi* (Record of Rites), compiled by Tai the Younger ca. Han dynasty 50 B.C. The earliest section may date from the time of the *Lun yu* (Digested Conversations) of *Confucian Analects* ca. 465-450 B.C.; translated by J. Legge, 1885; F. S. Couvreur, 1913; and R. Wilhelm, 1930.

k. *Ta tai li chi* (Record of Rites) compiled by Tai the Elder ca. Han dynasty between A.D. 80-100. Attributed editor is Tai Te, but in fact it was probably edited by Ts'ao Pao; translated by R. K. Douglas in 1882 and R. Wilhelm in 1930.

l. *Huai nan tzu* (The Book of the Prince of Huai Nan) ca. 120 B.C.

m. *Chi jan*. This is a fragment of a lost book dated ca. fifth century B.C. Chapter 9 entitled *"Fu Kuo"* (How to Make the Country Prosperous) was found in the *Wu yueh chuen chiu* (Spring and Autumn Annals of the States of Wu and Yueh). This chapter describes conversations between Chi Ni Tzu and Kou Chien, King of Yueh. Kou Chien asked his advisor his opinion about a contemplated invasion of the state of Wu. Chi Ni Tzu demurred and recommended that the king be more concerned about natural phenomena to increase agricultural resources and enrich the populace: "Yin must observe the *ch'i* of heaven and earth, trace the activities of the yin and the yang, and know the *Ku-hsu* (gate of heaven and the door of the earth). Yin must understand survival and death. Only then can yin weigh up your enemy." This advice was followed by great success. It is likely that the original was available to Chang.

n. *Chuen chiu fan lu* (String of Pearls in the Spring and Autumn Annals) by Tung Chung-shu ca. 135 B.C. Yin and yang are discussed as polar opposites in Chapter 57. Their relationships to heavan, earth, man, tao, *ch'i*, and *ching* are reviewed and their influence on disease mechanisms described.

Appendix 4

Books on Herbs (*Pen T'sao*)

The earliest *pen ts'ao* (pharmacopeia) *Shen-Nung pen ts'ao* is no longer in existence in its original form but is thought to have been written in the early Han period by the *Fang Shih,* a guild of magicians and technicians. (The guild included pharmacologists who were engaged in the search for the elixir of life.) Some of the material then was collected from Chou and Warring State data and added in the later Han era. The collection was given the name of the legendary Shen Nung, thus the title *Shen-Nung pen ts'ao.* Numerous copies appeared subsequently, often with additions, deletions, and errors. One of them was the *Lei-kung-chi-chu-Shen-Nung pen ts'ao,* now known only through descriptions found in other books such as *Cheng-lei pen ts'ao, T'ai-ping-yu-lan pen ts'ao* et al. The *Shen nung* originally appeared in four volumes. The first contained general information on herbs and the remaining books discussed medicine on three levels: volume two on the upper level — the elixir of life; volume three on the middle level — tonics for preserving health; and volume four on the lower level — curatives.

The medicines, many of which are widely used today, were largely vegetable in origin with some of mineral and animal origin.

The descriptions of a drug included its *ch'i* or temperature (*han* — cold; *je* — hot; *wen* — warm; *liang* — cool), its taste (*kan* — sweet; *suan* — sour; *hsin* — tart; *k'u* — bitter; and *hs'ien* — salty), its use and effectiveness, and synonyms.

In the Warring States (*Chan Kuo*) Period (480-221 B.C.) myths widely prevailed. The three most famous were "Peng-lai," "Fang-chang," and "In-chou." The main theme centered on the pursuit of drugs that would give man immortality. One of these legends tells that Chin Shih Huang Ti delegated Hsu Fu, along with several thousand young men and women in 219 B.C. to search for the dwellings of the immortals of the Eastern seas in the hope of finding the elixir of life. This goal was never achieved, but the group ended up in Japan, and probably introduced Chinese medicine to the Japanese. Others were dispatched subsequently in 215 B.C. — Master Lu, Han Chung, the venerable Hou, and Master Shih — with the same negative result. In the same year the emperor decreed that the naturalists should search out, select, and prepare wonderful medicines (*ch'i yao*), another example no doubt of his interest in finding the herb of eternal life. The above information was recorded faithfully in the *Shih chi* (Historical Records) ca. 90 B.C. by Ssu Ma Ch'ien and his father, Ssu Ma T'an.

Tao Hung-ching (A.D. 452-536), the great pharmacologist of the Tsin dynasty, compiled his *Shen Nung pen ts'ao ching* by using all the previous data, including the *Lei kung chi chu Shen Nung pen ts'ao*. His researches. written in three volumes, combined the *Shen nung pen ts'ao* and the *Ming i pieh lu.* The latter listed 365 drugs used by eminent physicians of the Han and Wei dynasties. Volume I consisted of an introduction to the *Shen nung pen ts'ao* with explanatory notes. Volume II and III discussed a total of 730 various herbs (365 from the original source and 365 from the *Ming i pieh lu*). The former were written in red and the latter in black for ready identification. Descriptions of the drugs included *chi* (taste), toxicity, synonyms, source, and methods of preparation. A natural classification system was used. Volume II discussed minerals, herbs, and trees; and Volume III, drugs of animal derivation and edibles, such as fruits, nuts, greens, and grains.

Tao divided 365 kinds of herbs into the following categories:

I.   Superior (imperial preparations): 120 kinds, usually

non-toxic tonics which promote health and comfort.

II. General herbal drugs (ministeral preparations): 120 kinds which were either toxic or non-toxic and used to treat mental diseases.

III. Inferior herbal drugs (assistant preparations): 125 which usually produced a toxic reaction and were recommended for the treatment of various disorders.

This ancient classification of Chinese herb medicine is somewhat like that of modern medicine in which drugs are divided into toxic and non-toxic categories.

Tao subsequently enlarged his original treatise from three to seven volumes. The first book remained unaltered, but the special *tse* material in Volumes II and III were extended to six volumes. None have survived but incomplete portions of Volume I and the section on animals. This material is reviewed here because some of the earlier information must have been available to Chang for study.

Some information on natural products may be found in the *Shih ching* or *Book of Odes* which Chang no doubt read. This is a work of ancient folk songs. Its author is unknown, but it has been dated to the Chou dynasty, which lasted from the ninth to the fifth century B.C.

The *Shan hai ching* (Classic of the Mountains and Seas) was in existence in Chang's times. The Shan portion was written ca. 400 B.C. and the Hai portion ca. 250 B.C. The two parts were combined subsequently; authors, unknown. It has been translated recently into English by Hui Chen-cheng et al. The *Shan ching* is a geography of China, particularly of the mountain ranges. Twenty-six of the chapters, which are arranged according to regions, have references in them to medicines. Three chapters cover the *Nan shan ching,* the south mountains; four, the *Hsi shan ching,* the west mountains; three, the *Pei shan ching,* the north mountains; four, the *Tung shan ching,* the east mountains; and twelve, the *Chung shan ching,* the central mountains. The material covered includes information on 270 animals, 70 minerals, and 150 plants, of which 47 animals and 21 plants are used as medicinals. Some examples are as follows: minerals – realgar and talc; animals – dragon bone, musk, *Bovis calculus, Cervi pantotrichum cornu;* plants – *Cinnamomi cortex, angelicae radix, Cnidii rhizoma,* platycodon, *Mori radicis cortex, Aurantii*

citrus, Aiayphus, Rubiae radix, Uncariae cum uncis ramulus.
The *Hai ching* does not contain any references to medicine.

Some comments on herbs and trees may be found in the *Erh ya,* an ancient dictionary dating from the Chou dynasty and discussed by Kuo-p'o (A.D. 276-324). This material was reviewed by E. Bretschneider in Volume II, *The Botany of the Chinese Classics,* (1892) of the three volumes of *Botanicum Sinicum.*

Hua To's (A.D. 110-207), a contemporary of Chang, work must have been available and familiar to Chang. His main interest was in surgery and anesthesia using *Ma-fei-san* (hemp), but he made contributions in other areas such as hydro-therapy, acupuncture, antiseptics, and anthelminthics.

Appendix 5

Books on the Pulse

The value of the pulse in diagnosis has been well established and was known in China in ancient times. Its use in the recognition of disease was recorded in the *Nei ching*. Pien Chüeh (Pien Ch'io, Chin Yueh Jen) who lived between 407 and 310 B.C. was also well versed in pulse lore. He made three significant contributions to medicine: (1) he standardized the methods of Chinese diagnosis -- observing, listening, questioning, and palpating the pulse and abdomen -- which remain in use to this day; (2) he wrote the *Nan ching*, a book on medical perplexities derived from the *Nei ching*; (3) he recorded perhaps the first clinical use of acupuncture in the treatment of the Prince of Chin. Note: The dates given above are commonly accepted although Ssu Ma Ch'ien in his *Shih chi* (Historical Records) fixes the only date known to be accurate for Pien Chueh as 501 B.C. when this celebrated physician is recorded as attending to an illness of a prince of Chin.

It is also quite likely that the work of Ch'un-Yu I (Shun-Yu I, Ts'ang Kung) was well known to Chang. His biography is also recorded in the *Shih chi* (Historical Records). He was born in 216 B.C. and died between 150 and 145 B.C. His main contribution was a detailed description of twenty-five clinical case histories, all of which have survived. The histories are of seventeen men, six women, and two children. Unfortunately the symptoms and signs of illness are poorly described, and although much stress was placed on pulse diagnosis, his notes are vague. Some of the problems encountered included gastric and genito-urinary disorders, rheumatism, toothache, tumors, paralysis, and hemoptysis. Herbal treatment was preferred with only occasional use of acupuncture and hydrotherapy. There were ten deaths. Ch'un was said to have had five students, all of whom are unknown. There are no further surviving writings with one additional exception which concerns his replies to a series of eight specific questions. These replies were in response to an imperial command given in 154 B.C. that he reveal the nature of his practice.

Ch'un-Yu I's teacher Yang Ch'ing, a pulse expert, gave him a book called *Mo shu shang hsia ching* (Treatise on the Pulse in Two Manuals). One manual was associated with the name of Pien Chüeh (Pien Ch'io), already mentioned, and the other with the name of Huang Ti. This manual could be a possible early form of the *Nei ching* as some of the chapters are quite similar in the *Mo shu shang hsu ching* and the *Nei ching*. Some of the similar chapters are *"Wu se chen"* (Diagnosis by the Five Colors); *"Ch'i kai shu"* (The Art of Determining the Loci of the Eight Auxiliary Tracts) about acupuncture; *"K'uei tu yin yang"* (The Determination of the Degree of Yin and Yang) about various diseases, *"Pien yao"* (Drugs Effecting Changes in the Body), and *"Lun shih"* (Discussion on the Use of Mineral Drugs).

Appendix 6
Malaria

Chang Chung-ching was undoubtedly aware of the disease that we now know as malaria. The name "malaria" is derived from the colloquial Italian *mala* meaning bad and *aria* meaning "air". The term first appeared in English literature about 1829, it being supposed that the disease was due to poisonous emanations from damp ground. The disease was also known to Hippocrates (460-370 B.C.) who described it as "periodic fevers" in his *Book of Epidemics*. He divided the fevers into quotidian, tertian, quartan, and subtertian types and noted the presence of splenomegaly (an enlarged spleen). Celsus also discussed two types of tertian fever in the first century: one benign, similar to quartan fever; the other, more severe with a longer duration, the fever persisting for thirty-six or forty-eight hours, never completely subsiding but recurring in remissions. The disease is now known to be due to protozoan parasites of the class sporozoa of the genus *Plasmodium*. The parasites were first identified by Alphonse Laveran on November 6, 1880, at Constantine, Algeria, and their mosquito transmission proposed by Sir Patrick Manson in 1894.

Sir Ronald Ross became acquainted with Manson when

he was on leave to England from the Indian Medical Service in 1894. Convinced of the truth of the mosquito origin of malaria, Ross returned to Indian and carried on his research from 1895-1899, all the while communicating with Manson. His work was done on a malarial disease of sparrows due to *Plasmodium praecox*. Ross was able to infect 22 out of 28 healthy sparrows by mosquitoes of the genus *Culex* which had fed previously on sparrows ill with the disease. The complete cycle of development of the parasite was observed in the culicine mosquito which was used for transmission. The cycle of transmission and infection was later demonstrated in humans infected by the anopheline mosquito (*Anopheles maculipennis*) by G. B. Grassi, a professor of zoology, and A. Bignami, a physician, both of Rome, Italy. Ross received the Nobel prize in medicine on December 10, 1902 for his distinguished accomplishment.

Malaria in man is caused by the following *Plasmodia*:

    P. falciparum (malignant tertian, subtertian, or *falciparum* malaria)

    P. vivax (benign tertian malaria or *vivax* malaria)

    P. malariae (quartan malaria or *malariae* malaria)

    P. ovale (*ovale* tertian malaria or *ovale* malaria)

Mixed infections may occur. The most common and important of these infections are those due to *P. falciparum* and *P. ovale*.

Modern treatment of malaria is directed towards the eradication or control of the parasite and treatment of the complications. The clinical picture of the disease is produced by erythrocytic invasion by the parasite. Effective control can be achieved only by their removal and by the anti-inflammatory activity of the medication prescribed. Drugs which act on the blood level are called schizonticides. Chloroquine (or some other 4-amino quinoline), quinine, mepacrine, proguanil, and pyrimethamine are the commonly used preparations which successfully control the condition in most regions. The first three have an anti-inflammatory activity. Quinine is not very effective and mepacrine is now seldom used. Primaquine and pamaquine are 8-amino quinolines. They are weak schizonticides but quite helpful in controlling the tissue forms of parasites such as those that infect the liver. Suppressive doses of proguanil, mepacrine, and chloroquine may lead to a radical cure in *falciparum* malaria, but in other types there is a tendency toward relapse after treatment is completed. Prophylactic therapy with all drugs is advised immediately on entering an endemic area and should be continued for some time after leaving. The only exception is the drug mepacrine which must be taken two weeks in advance.

Appendix 7
Jaundice

Jaundice

Jaundice (icterus) is a yellowish staining of the skin, mucous membranes, and certain body fluids by bile pigments, commonly referred to as bilirubin. It is usually due to a disorder of the liver or biliary tract but may result also from an excessive breakdown of hemoglobin within the body. It has been found also in some cases of myxedema and in individuals who have ingested large amounts of carrots, tomatoes, oranges, squash, spinach, egg yolk, or other sources of dietary pigmentation (carotene).

Jaundice may be obstructive or medical (hepatogenous) in origin.

1. *Obstructive jaundice*. This type results from any obstruction of the normal flow of bile in the biliary system. One cause is carcinoma of the pancreas, gall bladder, bile ducts, or liver which often results in a complete obstruction of the vital organs and may or may not be amenable to surgery. Varying degrees of obstruction may be due also to congenital malformations of the bile ducts, cholangitis, cholangiolitis, and calculi, all of which may also indicate surgery.

2. *Medical jaundice*. There is also a variety of medical or

hepatogenous jaundice caused by such various things as viral-infectious hepatitis or acute or sub-acute liver atrophy. Protozoal jaundice comes from Weil's disease, malaria, leishmaniasis, amebiasis, relapsing fever, etc; bacterial jaundice from thypoid fever, tuberculosis, pneumonia, mycotic-histoplasmosis, etc; metazoal jaundice from schistosomiasis and other liver flukes; and toxic jaundice from chlorinating hydrocarbons, sulfonamides, para-amino-salicylic acid, and some antibiotics.

Laboratory tests

The following tests are often helpful in differentiating jaundice.

Prothrombin time shows malabsorption of Vitamin K, commonly seen with extrahepatic cholestasis.

Transaminase shows if the serum glutamic oxaloacetic transaminase (SGOT) is greater than 5,600 U.; if so the jaundice is most likely due to hepatitis.

Serum alkaline phosphatase tests are helpful in diagnosing cases of viral and alcoholic hepatitis, as well as mechanical obstruction.

Serum bilirubin is examined to determine any characteristic change.

Serum protein can be tested with electrophoretic methods.

Serum immunoglobulins indicate parenchymal liver disease.

Hepatitis B antigen, alpha fetoglobulin, and *carcinoembryonic antigen* tests show type B hepatitis.

X-rays-routine, KUB, cholangiography, or radionucleotides of the kidneys, ureters, and bladder also will indicate hepatitis.

An *endoscopy, liver biopsy,* or *exploratory laparotomy* are other methods by which jaundice can be diagnosed.

Appendix 8
Worm Infestation

There would appear to be little doubt that the descriptions concerning patients vomiting worms refer to the modern classification of Nematoda or round worms. In this particular instance, the most common type would fall into the categorization of the intestinal roundworm *Ascaris lumbricoides*. This is one of the most common helminthic infections (especially children), known to man. Infection occurs usually by swallowing embryonated ova that are present in soil, water, vegetables, and other types of food. Liberated in the small intestine, the larvae penetrate the intestinal wall, migrate to the mesentric lymphatics and venules, and are then carried through the right side of the heart to the lungs. After a few days they break through the pulmonary capillaries into the air sacs, at which time the patient coughs up bloody sputum which is reswallowed and passed again to the small intestine where the worms attain maturity in eight to ten weeks. Eggs are extruded in the stools; and if fertilized, develop vermicules which are infective if swallowed. Vomiting of these round worms may occur as described by Chang. An infection of round worms may result in malnutrition, eosinophilia (only as allergic reaction to the worms), and/or intestinal obstruction.

An effective modern treatment is piperazine salts (citrate, adipate, or phosphate) in single doses of 4 gm followed by a saline purge the next day. A syrup is available for children. Bephenium hydroxynaphthoate (alcopar), which is effective in hookworm infestion, is also useful in ascariasis. The adult dose is 2.5 gm with half this amount given to children under two years of age. The treatment is continued for three days when there is diarrhea.

Infections of hookworms, also classified with the nematodes, include *Ancylostoma duodenale* and *Necator americanus* which are not uncommon and are usually associated with unsanitary conditions. Eggs are passed through the feces and develop into the sheathed filariform larvae which infect man by penetrating the skin. They migrate to the right ventricle of the heart, thence to the lungs and alveoli, and are finally swallowed. They then reach the intestinal tract where the cycle is repeated. Expectoration of blood, vomiting of worms, malaise, dyspnea, loss of appetite, digestive disturbances, edema, and pallor are commonly present. Besides there may also be tachycardia, an enlarged flabby heart, heart failure, and malnutrition with retarded growth and development in childhood. Anemia, eosinophilia, and hypoalbuminenia may also be present.

The diagnosis of hookworms is usually made, as in all worm infestations, by recovery and identification of the eggs in the feces. Treatment includes correction of the anemia and use of anthelminthics. Tetracycline in a dosage of 0.1 ml/kg body weight with a maximum dose of 5 ml is given in the morning on an empty stomach. Bephenium hydroxynaphthoate (alcopar) is more effective in treating *Ancylostoma duodenale* in a dosage of 5 gm repeated for three consecutive days. Bitoscanate (Jonit Phenylene diiosothyocyanate 1,4) is used in 100 mg doses b.i.d., p.c. and repeated on the next morning only. Thiabendazole (mintezol) is used in 250 mg/kg body weight b.i.d. doses for two days for cases of mixed infections of ascaris and hookworm. Other effective drugs include Pyrantel pamoate (combantrin), tetramizole, and mebendazole.

Another common worm infestation, probably also known by Chang, is due to *Strongyloides stercoralis*. The larvae are passed in human feces and grow in the soil into free-living adults.

These pierce the human skin, migrate to the right side of the heart, penetrate the pulmonary vessels, and pass into the alveoli. If they are swallowed, vomiting may result, but many reach the intestinal tract and the cycle is repeated. The clinical picture is quite similar to that observed in hookworm infestation with symptoms of abdominal pain, nausea, vomiting, and diarrhea or constipation. The symptoms mimic duodenal ulcer. Occasionaly there is hematemesis, diarrhea with tenesmus, and bloody stools. Skin reactions may also be present. For treatment Thisbendazole is the most effective drug and is given in doses of 25 mg/kg body weight b.i.d. for two or three days.

Appendix 9
Cholera

Cholera

Although cholera as such was unknown to Chang Chung-ching, apparently there was a similar disease, maybe the same disease, existing in his time.

Cholera is an acute, often fatal, infectious disease of short duration caused by a specific organism: *Vibrio cholerae* (*Spirillum cholerae*). It was discovered by Robert Koch in 1883. The organism multiplies in the bowel but does not invade the blood stream or tissues. Cholera is characterized by profuse watery diarrhea, vomiting, muscular cramps, suppression of urine, severe dehydration, and vascular collapse. It is endemic in origin and associated with poverty and poor sanitation.

Cholera, symptomatically, can be divided into two stages as a result of the proliferation of the comma bacillus in the small intestine in conjunction with a liberation of toxins.

1. The state of evacuation lasts two to twelve hours and exhibits severe diarrhea which rapidly assumes a rice-water appearance, prostration, vomiting -- retching often tinged with blood, hiccoughs, agonizing muscle cramps, cyanosis, loss of body fluids with typical cholera facies, an initial increase then de-

crease in heartbeat, unquenchable thirst, oliguria, and a decrease in surface temperature, along with a mild elevation of the rectal temperature.

2. The algid stage or stage of collapse is characterized by signs of circulatory failure: fast, almost imperceptible pulse (120-160); cold and clammy skin; weak voice; frequent cessation of purging and vomiting; a decrease in blood pressure; rapid and shallow respirations with subsequent respiratory failure; asthenia; coma; and eventually death. The patient's appearance is cadaveric but the mental faculties remain until the end.

Not withstanding, the recovery rate is high when effective therapy is employed except in the more critically involved patient and those in shock.

The diagnosis is made in patients who present the following symptoms:

1. a sudden onset of vomiting
2. profuse diarrhea
3. extreme prostration
4. circulatory collapse
5. cholera facies
6. painful muscle cramps
7. urinary suppression

The diagnosis is relatively easy to make in epidemics although any medical problem resulting in acute dehydration, vomiting, and watery diarrhea may stimulate cholera, including algid falciparum malaria, heat exhaustion, and acute food or chemical poisoning.

History

References to cholera in early Western literature are indefinite. Thucydides, the Greek historian (460-401 B.C.), described in *Book II,* Sec. 47-53-54, an epidemic disease that was manifested by severe, watery diarrhea and marked asthenia resulting in considerable mortality among the Athenians. Hippocrates (460-377 B.C.), the father of Western medicine, known for his many treatises, is remembered particularly for his system of ethics and morality embodied in the well known "Hippocratic Oath" taken by all Western physicians on graduating from medical college. Yet even he did not clearly define the condition of cholera as we know it today.

Susruta (ca. 1000 B.C.), the father of Indian surgery, discusses both medical and surgical problems in his *Medical Compendium* which was intended for students of medicine. He described a disease that manifested vomiting, diarrhea, pain, cyanosis of the legs and nails, a weak voice, and a sinking in of the eyes--all of which were probably due to cholera. There would appear to be little doubt that the disease has been endemic in India for centuries, resulting in periodic epidemics which occasionally reach pandemic proportions. There are many published accounts of cholera in the world literature from the sixteenth century onward. Some investigators have propounded that true cholera did not reach China from India until 1669. However, a severe epidemic did reach China from India by the land route in 1817, and subsequent outbreaks have since been well documented in modern literature.

Western literature on the early history of cholera in China has been summarized by Wong and Wu. It is unfortunate that many of their references cannot be checked for additional details as they are buried in Chinese customs and Protestant missionary society records not now readily available.

Dudgeon in the "Customs Medical Report," No. 4, p. 39, 1872 as recorded by Wong and Wu on page 384, footnote 371, and on pages 384-389 refers to the history and belief in the antiquity of cholera. He states that it was described as early as 2500 B.C. as "*hua luan*" by which name it is still known today. The expression means something huddled up in a confused manner inside the body which is evidenced by the vomiting and purging. He quotes several ancient Chinese writers (not included by Wong and Wu) but states there was no mention of its epidemic character.

Wong and Wu refer to the work of Su-tzemi without quoting the reference, but their discussion of his short article gives a description of the cholera epidemic of 1812 which appeared in Kiahsing on the borders of Chekiang and Kiangsu. Su-tzemi felt that cholera was a new disease and described it as "contracting the leg tendons disease" (tiao chiao sha). He felt the disease to be due to "morbific cold" and recommended warming or stimulating the vessels. He also pointed out that occasionally no distinction was made between cholera and gastroenteritis.

David Manson also felt that there was evidence in Fukien annals that cholera existed in epidemic form before the nineteenth century and that the first outbreak of this type occurred in Fukien in 1812.

Macgowan also questioned whether cholera was a new disease (Wang and Wu, text, page 384; footnote 373, page 386) in his 1881 Wenchow report, but he admits the possibility in a subsequent paper written in 1883-1884.

Simmons (Wong and Wu, pgs. 386 and 387 and footnote 378, page 386) reported instances of earlier epidemics in the eighteenth century. He felt that this pestilence was usually imported because the Chinese had a habit of drinking boiled water or tea and their method of disposal of night soil (sewerage) tended to localize and keep any infection in check whereas in India there was a complete absence of cleansing rites for drinking or bathing in the rivers and lakes connected with pilgrimmages.

Vaccinations with dead vibrios is obligatory for all individuals who are within or may enter an endemic area. This provides partial protection for three months even though the current international certificate of vaccination is valid for six months. It usually reduces the incidence of the disease in approximately 50 percent of the cases although it can still occur in an individual who has had repeated inoculations.

Treatment

There is no specific treatment for cholera. However, it is mandatory to rehydrate the individual with intravenous saline transfusions; to correct the acidosis with transfusions of solutions containing sodium bicarbonate or lactate; to restore electrolyte balance (particularly potassium); and to institute measures to control oligemic shock and uremic anuria.

Infusions with saline are helpful in controlling hypotension, and corticosteroids and L-noradrenaline are therapeutic for patients in shock. The addition of 5 to 10 percent glucose to the transfusion is helpful for those who are comatose, particularly children. Mepyramine and related drugs are used for the vomiting. Analgesics relieve the severe pain and muscular cramps but morphine is contraindicated. Tetany is relieved by calcium gluconate given intravenously.

Antibiotics, particularly tetracycline, help to reduce the volume and duration of the evacuations. Tetracycline is given in doses of 250 mg. every six hours for forty-eight hours and is started three hours after replacement treatment has been instituted and vomiting controlled. Chloramphenicol has a similar effect but tetracycline is preferred.

Index

(Boldface numbers indicate pages where
formulas' compositions are detailed)

A

B

C

ABOUT THE AUTHORS

Dr. Keisetsu Otsuka (1900-1980) graduated from Kumamoto Medical College and studied Chinese herbal medicine under Yumoto Kyushin. He practiced as a Chinese herbal physician from 1931 until his death in 1980. One-time president of the Medical Association of Japan, in 1972 he directed the Comprehensive Oriental Research Institute, affiliated with the Kitasato Institute.

Dr. Hong-yen Hsu earned his Doctor of Pharmacy degree at the University of Kyoto. He remained in Japan for three more years as a member of the research staff at the University of Tokyo. Since 1945 he has actively engaged in teaching and research at National Taiwan University and the medical colleges in Taipei, Taichung, and Kaohsiung, and has served as acting chief of the Taiwan Provincial Hygienic Laboratory, director of the Food and Drug Control Bureau, dean of the Botany Department at the Chinese Culture University, director of the Institute of Pharmacological Science at the China Medical College, and president of the Brion Research Institute of Taiwan. He founded the Oriental Healing Arts Institute in 1976.

William G. Peacher, M.D., has a distinguished background in neurology, neurosurgery, speech pathology, psychology and rehabilitation medicine. He spent considerable time in advanced studies of herbal medicine and acupuncture in Europe and Asia and has substantially assisted the efforts of the Oriental Healing Arts Institute. Instrumental in establishing licensure of Oriental medicine through the New York State Board of Medicine (1974-1975), he has maintained his interest in the field since moving to California in 1978.

Handel Wu, a pharmacist graduated from Taipei Medical College, has been working as an English secretary at the Brion Research Institute of Taiwan for many years.

Wang Su-yen, also a pharmacist graduated from Taipei Medical College, is now director of the translation and compilation division of the Brion Research Institute of Taiwan.